AWESOME
AFTER FORTY

Advanced Praise for
Awesome After Forty

With decades of experience in strength, fitness, and nutrition, Cliff and Daz focus less on looks or competition and more on building lasting resilience and function. They cover the essentials: smart training that prioritises strength and quality movement, real food nutrition that adapts to your lifestyle, and the often-overlooked pillars of sleep and stress. With down-to-earth advice on injury prevention, chronic pain, and easy self-checks, this book gives everyone the tools to keep performing well and enjoying life for decades to come.

Dr Mikki Williden

Nutritionist/Researcher

I've known Daz for nearly 20 years, and what has always stood out to me is the heart and integrity he brings to everything he does. His experience and expertise in programming, movement, and nutrition advice had a huge impact on me. Under his guidance, I became fitter, stronger, and mentally tougher than at any other point in my athletic career, even as an ageing athlete.

But what makes Daz special is helping people see the value of strength and movement in everyday life and giving them confidence to carry that into everything they do.

This book gives you a glimpse of the guy we've all been lucky to learn from, and why his influence sticks with you.

Jenny May Clarkson

Silver Fern/TV Presenter

Cliff and Darren's book is an inspiring and genuinely helpful guide for anyone wanting to stay fit, healthy, and energised beyond forty. Their insights are practical, grounded in real experience and science, and delivered with honesty and warmth. I have known Cliff for many years, and he is living proof of his own message — he truly walks the walk as well as talks the talk — and this authenticity shines through. It's a refreshing take on what it means to age well, not just physically, but with purpose and vitality.

I'm inspired to lift my game!

Scott Gooding

Personal Trainer/Chef

Cliff and Darren have pooled years of knowledge and experience to create a brilliant handbook for anyone wanting to achieve optimal health as they age. Full of practical health info and instruction that is informed by the most current science. Such a great book.

Art Green
Personal Trainer/TV Presenter

AWESOME
AFTER FORTY

Time-tested Strength, Nutrition, and Lifestyle techniques to be healthy, happy, and strong after 40

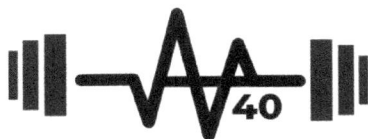

CLIFF HARVEY PhD & DARREN ELLIS MSc

KATOA HEALTH PUBLISHING | AUCKLAND, NEW ZEALAND

ISBN 978-1-0671209-0-0 (Paperback)

ISBN 978-1-0671209-1-7 (EPUB)

Katoa Health Publishing (a division of Holistic Performance Limited)

Disclaimer: The information in this book is for educational purposes only and is not intended as a substitute for professional medical advice. The authors and publisher are not liable for any injuries or damages that may result from the use of this book's content. Always consult with a qualified healthcare provider before beginning any new fitness or nutrition program.

Contents

FOREWORD

By Dr Eric Helms

As I write this, I'm one week out from stepping on a World Natural Bodybuilding Federation (WNBF) pro stage. At forty-two years old, with twenty-one years of lifting—half my life—under my belt, I am in the best shape of my life. This isn't an exaggeration; it's the objective reality.

Next week, I will compete against the best natural bodybuilders on the planet, a privilege I fought for throughout my twenties but only achieved in 2023, the year I turned forty. Today, I stand at the peak of my athletic career, a living testament to a simple truth: your forties are not an epilogue to your youth; they can be the beginning of your prime. The principles that made this possible are encapsulated in the book you are about to read.

I can think of no two individuals better equipped to guide you on this journey than Dr Cliff Harvey and Darren Ellis. I have had the pleasure of calling these men my friends and colleagues for the thirteen years since I moved to New Zealand. I've shared stages with Cliff at presentations around the world, worked alongside them both at the Holistic Performance Institute, and spent countless hours talking shop about lifting and life. Cliff and I even navigated our doctoral studies together at AUT. Before that, back in 2012, when I was a master's student on a tight budget, it was Cliff who generously provided the protein powder that made my research financially feasible.

You couldn't find two gentlemen more pragmatic, kind, and generous, whose decades of practical, in-the-trenches experience are perfectly balanced by their scientific training and academic backgrounds. They don't just talk the talk; they have walked it, and they have helped thousands of others do the same.

The power of this book lies in its focus on the "big rocks"—the foundational pillars that create real, lasting change. Cliff and Daz correctly emphasise training coordinated movement patterns over simply training muscles. While my current focus is bodybuilding—this year marks my 20th show—it's a specialisation I've only undertaken in the last four years, born from an acceptance that I'm more competitive at *looking* strong than *being* strong. This focus, however, is built on a broad foundation.

From 2006 to 2021, I was a multi-sport athlete, competing in 20 powerlifting meets, five weightlifting meets, two strongman competitions, and a highland games competition. This background embodies the timeless ideal of physical culture, where strength, health, and aesthetics go hand in hand, as exemplified by the champions of the past like John Grimek and Tommy Kono. My "Why" is rooted in this identity as a lifelong lifter. It's why I will likely return to the powerlifting platform in the future, swapping my posing trunks for a lifting singlet, with a very realistic goal of being at my strongest ever, even in my mid-to-late forties. By adopting this long-term, holistic view, there is no "on" or "off" switch. Adherence is not a matter of willpower; it's a matter of being the person I envision myself to be and aligning my actions with my values.

This message has never been more important or timely. Men over forty are constantly bombarded with narratives of frailty and decline. We're told we've "lost a step," and that the only solution is to recapture our youth with testosterone replacement therapy or other quick fixes that have us looking backwards. This book provides a powerful counter-narrative, one grounded in reality. The data and real-world evidence show that men in their forties and fifties can still be in their physical prime. Much of what we associate with ageing is simply the cumulative effect of inactivity, unintentional eating, and, most critically, letting the busyness of adult life disconnect us from our values and our "Why."

Cliff and Daz have created more than a training manual; they've written a charter for thriving in what can and should be the most awesome chapter of your life. I wholeheartedly endorse this book. Read it, apply its principles, and get ready to redefine what's possible.

Dr Eric Helms

Senior Research Fellow, AUT/WNBF Professional Bodybuilder

INTRODUCTION

Why We Wrote This Book

Cliff: ***I pulled 360 kg (836 lb) from the rack.*** *It wasn't easy and it wasn't hard, but there wasn't any more room left on the bar to stack on more weights. It also wasn't particularly 'pretty' as lifts go, but hey, it got up there (and that's all that matters, right?) …*

Stepping out of the rack, I felt a sharp pain in my back, and my knees instantaneously gave way. I hit the floor, but strangely, when I got up, the pain, while still 'there', was just a dull ache around my lower back and left hip. Little did I know that this seminal event in my early 30s would set me on a decade-long journey into injury, debility, and eventually recovery…

You're probably reading this because you are either a former athlete trying to recover or maintain your condition as you age, someone who's never trained before (but knows that you need to do 'something' to live better and longer), or you're an 'old dog' athlete still grinding away trying to maintain performance and health for the long term.

Unfortunately, we accept that as we age, we will inevitably experience degeneration. We make excuses for ourselves by saying "I'm not what I used to be" or "I'm just getting old." I've wondered, though, many times through the years, just how much degeneration should we accept? While some degree of peak performance will be lost as we age (that's why we don't see 80-year-old running backs in the NFL), does that mean that we need to accept becoming weak, sick, and tired? And what's the deal with 40?

While in previous generations, 40 might have marked a more significant turning point in one's life, nowadays, it seems arbitrary to accept that we'll become markedly less functional once we're 'over the hill' at 40.

My goal with this book is to introduce you to sustainable and effective strategies and tactics for achieving strength, health, and a life well-lived. Thankfully, I have as my co-author a legend in the fields of functional fitness, strength, and nutrition, my good buddy Darren 'Daz' Ellis.

Daz: While a large part of my fitness journey involved the same vulnerability of injury Cliff experienced, I wanted to mention some other aspects of the 'fitness-industrial complex' I encountered over the years.

In 2015, I was the fittest 40-year-old in Australasia, qualifying as the second fittest worldwide to compete at The CrossFit Games. I worked my butt off daily to get stronger, to be faster, to go for longer. Yet I didn't really feel *fit* in the way I personally defined it. Despite the 'constant variance' of CrossFit, I missed the ocean swimming, paddleboarding and mountain biking I used to do, I missed the play – tumbling, climbing, balancing, etc....it's funny how so many people talk about CrossFit being dangerous, because when I was approaching a competition, I would avoid going out on my bike for fear of hurting myself!

It was becoming difficult for me to enjoy training because the whole reason I started was to use that training to get outside, express my fitness and explore the natural world. Instead, I was effectively working out to get better at working out...

Don't get me wrong, that was an acceptable sacrifice at the time, but what really hit home was realising how many of my clients wanted to pursue this same sacrifice. I felt so torn, wanting to support their dreams, when deep down I knew that the majority (who had stressful jobs, families, and long injury histories) would be so much better off eliminating joint pain, getting more sleep, increasing functional strength, and losing some body fat.

More importantly, while the pursuit of increased performance is important for significant progress, to do so at the exclusion of all things (social, recreational, travel, etc.) results in an unbalanced and potentially unhealthy way to get fit.

For the past few years, when talking to gym owners, coaches, and athletes, the same issues have been coming up for them. But when I talked about what I was doing, their eyes would glaze over... The 'cool' elements of fitness are very entrenched – the intensity, the big weights, gruelling workouts, embracing 'the grind'...

Exercise has become 'exertainment' instead of a place for purpose and growth. I knew that it was going to be a relearning process for many and that it would be difficult, but I also knew that sustainable programming and training practices are the solution to poor movement, injuries, and lack of progress. Just lately, the effects of the COVID-19 pandemic have led to an increased awareness of, and readiness to embrace a less-is-more approach.

And so, here we are...

You don't need to be stronger than a powerlifter, you just need to be stronger than the other dads...

Play on a quote from Pavel

What Makes You Awesome After 40?

Cliff: My take on how to be awesome after 40 is quite simple: it's to maintain generally the same capacity you had in your 20s and 30s (assuming you were in good health and fitness!) and be able to engage in a wide variety of movements and activities. It also means having a clear mind and a happy mood, being pain-free, and most importantly, being *functional* and able to *perform* well in all your daily activities.

Functional though is an overused and typically misapplied word. Many in the fitness industry have adopted the term "functional" to describe training that relies on balance devices, such as Bosu balls and stability balls, or odd objects, or hyper-specific training for sports or daily-life movements. While some of these concepts have their place (especially odd-object lifting), they are not 'functional' per se. Functional in physical health and fitness relates to the primary and tertiary definitions of the word – *useful* and *performing a particular function or operation.* So, when we talk about functional, we're really describing *transferability*, which is a more apt term.

Transferability refers to the benefits that your training provides for both your daily life and your athletic performance. Given that we all have limited time and energy, the efficacy of transferability denotes what is *most* functional. That might all sound a little complex, but an analogy from the fitness industry of the late 90s and 2000s describes this well.

In the 90s and through the first decade of the 2000s, trainers became enamoured with the use of stability balls, Bosu balls, and other instability devices. It was claimed that they were more 'functional' because by providing instability, they recruited more 'stabilising' (typically tonic) muscles and muscle patterns and therefore had a greater crossover to general life, sports performance, and long-term health.

However, it was found that benefits to stability, postural control, and core activation were gained equally effectively from standard, compound strength movements, such as squats, deadlifts, lunges, presses, cleans, and snatches (the 'meat and potatoes' of strength training), when performed on a stable surface. These movements also provided the added benefit of increased strength, speed, and power compared to instability training, due to the lower loads that can be lifted on an unstable surface. So, while instability was touted as being more functional (and it does have its uses, albeit limited), it was, in fact, less transferable and less effective than traditional strength training —and thus, less *functional*.

Living with the same (or as close to) functional capacity as your 20–30-year-old self requires attention to not just exercise, but also to sleep, stress management, mindfulness, media exposure, and nutrition. So, a holistic approach, backed by evidence, and considering the shifting demands of life as an over-40 athlete, is required.

Daz: I have always looked at this similarly to Cliff, reaching the pinnacle of my physical performance at the age of 40 (competing at the CrossFit Games). It was there, in black and white, proof that I had more going on than my 30-year-old self, and even my 20-year-old self. But once that lofty goal was attained, I immediately wondered, 'Could I be fitter at 50 than 40?'

Possibly...

What about 60?

At some point, everyone can see that this is not linear progress. Human life (and thus performance) is finite, so at some point, the peak will be reached.

The Latin phrase, 'Memento mori,' reminds us to 'remember, you will die.' Unfortunately, I see far too many people taking an approach to their fitness that indicates they believe in immortality!

The first step to being awesome after 40 is acceptance of where you are.

That does NOT mean you have to be satisfied. The beauty of fitness is that there are so many ways to practice and explore it. If you have maxed out your deadlift one-repetition maximum (1RM – the absolute most you can lift), that doesn't mean you can't keep making progress on the Romanian, Jefferson or single-leg deadlift.

If you can't match your marathon time from 10 years ago, what about trail runs? Adventure races? What about a 5-day Great Walk with loved ones?

We are all apprentices in a craft, in which no one becomes a master

Ernest Hemingway

01

START WITH *YOUR* ‘WHY’?

Why do you want to be healthy?

This might seem like a stupid question because *everyone* wants to be healthy, right? You might be tempted to skip past this section to the meaty stuff... but hold on, big fella...

Understanding your ‘why’ is a critical part of setting the right goals — not just any old goal — and finding the best path toward them. We often recognise that *something* in our lives isn’t quite right (a ‘pain-point’), or we feel that we lack direction and purpose. Therefore, we strive to find a solution to our problem and establish goals and objectives to enhance our lives. All of this is very laudable, but simply having a solution doesn’t make it the *right* solution, and merely having goals doesn’t make them the right goals; ones that are congruent with our ultimate, 'best-case' life of passion and purpose (one that meshes with our deepest ethos and values).

Now, if that all seems a little 'woo,' consider that we are far more likely to stick with health habits if we can emotionally connect to them and they align with our ethos and values.

In short, if you want to get the most out of your life and live in the best state of health, it's critical to start with your WHY?

With clients, I use a '3 Whys Exercise'.

The 3 'whys' exercise

Step 1. Brainstorm

- Get a big piece of paper and brainstorm all the reasons why you want to be 'healthy'
- Refine these ideas into a shortlist before moving on to Step 2.
- Make sure that the items on your shortlist are: **Personal, Positive, and Personally** compelling to you.

Step 2. Find your WHYs

On a piece of paper or in a document or sheet, put five columns and go through the following steps:

1. In the first column, put your list of whys
2. Go through the list one by one. Ask yourself why you want to achieve *that* why
3. Write your answer down in column 2
4. Now ask yourself why you want to achieve ***that*** why...
5. Write your answer in column 3
6. Repeat so that you have asked yourself 'why' at least 3 times
7. Now repeat these steps for each 'why'

By repeatedly asking ourselves why, we begin to delve deeper into our true reasons for doing something. Instead of just finding a why (or in other words, a reason) for doing things and *being* how we are, we can explore further and find the *true* reasons why we want to be healthy, not just the surface-level ones.

Step 3. Define key terms, concepts, and learnings

After completing the '3 levels of why' exercise, list some of the key learnings, terms, or concepts from each 'why'.

Note: these may not always be exactly related to the more 'concrete' things you have written in columns 1-4. Columns 1-4 serve as thought-starters, and by the time you have spent some time thinking, you will produce ideas that hint at your deeper ethos and values.

Step 4. Identify your personal health ethos

From column 5, pick 3-5 key concepts that define the most important outcomes for your life. These are your *personal health ethos*, a guiding set of principles that describe your ultimate **why.**

Ethos
A Greek word meaning "character" that is used to describe the guiding beliefs or ideals that characterise an ideology.

You may be surprised by what comes up, and it might significantly impact how you train, eat, and manage your life. For example, suppose you had an inkling that you might achieve your health goals by running a marathon, and yet, through this exercise, you identified that you wanted to spend a LOT more time with your family and also be a heck of a lot stronger. In that case, that goal may not be the correct one for you, and you might instead benefit from a health regimen centred around strength and minimum effective dose training (more on that later).

02

ASSESSMENT

Where are you now?

Having assessed your 'why,' you should have a better idea of what your optimal state of health, function, and fitness is, and most importantly, what it means to your life, and what tactics and strategies you need to apply for health.

This may have even drastically shifted your expectation of where you want to 'be' in life and health. So, you should have a good idea about whether your primary goal is to be bigger, leaner, stronger, 'fitter,' have more energy, or some combination of these or other health outcomes.

What do you *need* to do & be?

Knowing your why and where you want to be doesn't always define what you should do right now! There are critical components of overall 'fitness' that allow for not just the best outcomes for quality and length of life but also serve as the foundation to achieve your health and fitness goals, whatever they are.

Understanding where you're at *right now* will help define what you need to focus on to achieve your ultimate health. Unfortunately, however, many assessment protocols for health and fitness are overly complicated or require extensive time and financial investment. Thankfully, they are also unnecessary.

A few practical and straightforward assessments that you can carry out at home can identify which areas of health and fitness you should focus on.

The key physical assessments we'll be focusing on are:

Assessment	Domain measured	Training focus	Standard
Resting heart rate	Cardiometabolic health	Body composition, Strength, or Conditioning	< 67 beats per minute
Waist-height ratio	Cardiometabolic health	Body composition	Waist-to-height 0.5:1
Squat sit	Flexibility	Mobility	Able to hold a deep squat sitting position

Standing toe touch	Flexibility	Mobility	Ability to touch the toes in a standing position with legs straight
Pushup	Muscular endurance	Conditioning	40 repetitions
Farmers carry	Strength-endurance	Strength	30 seconds carrying 100% of bodyweight
Goblet squat with 50% of bodyweight	Muscular endurance	Conditioning	20 repetitions
Plank	Muscular endurance	Conditioning	2 minutes
Pullup	Strength	Strength	10 repetitions
Handstand pushup	Muscular strength	Strength	>1 full repetition
Deadlift	Muscular strength	Strength	150% bodyweight
Standing long jump	Power	Explosivity	Equivalent to your height
One leg stands for time	Balance	Strength	At least 45 seconds (eyes open) and 15 seconds (eyes closed)

In addition to the tests above, there are two factors with well-established associations with long-term health outcomes: residual movement (i.e., steps per day) and sleep.

Additional 'health-span'/lifestyle measures

- Monthly (per day) step average: 7000+
- Monthly sleep average: 7+hrs

How 'healthy' are you?

Basic Tests of Cardiometabolic Health

What is cardiometabolic health?

You've heard of cardiovascular health...heck, you may even know what it means – the health of the heart and circulatory system and vessels. *Cardiometabolic* takes this concept one step further and refers to not just the health of the heart and blood vessels but also to your overall metabolic health, especially blood sugar and insulin regulation, adiposity (body fat and body composition), and inflammatory and oxidative status, all of which affect overall health, risk of disease, and long-term mortality risk.

Testing for health is often overcomplicated. While extensive testing can be useful, far more accessible and, in most cases, more useful are a few simple tests that you can do at home.

Resting Heart Rate

Resting heart rate (RHR) is how many times your heart beats per minute at rest. Higher resting heart rates indicate lower cardiovascular fitness and a greater risk of cardiac dysfunction, atherosclerosis, and other conditions. It's not so much that a higher heart rate *causes* health problems, but more so that it is an excellent indicator that your diet, exercise, and lifestyle aren't 'on point' to preserve your cardiovascular and total health.

Higher resting heart rates compared to lower ones are associated with around a 50% increase in heart disease and cancer risks. Each 10 beats per minute (BPM) increase is associated with ~15% greater risk of these conditions, and every 10 BPM increase is associated with a 17% increased risk of death.[1]

How to perform the test

If you have a smartwatch, it will provide you with your resting heart rate. If you don't have a smartwatch, you can manually test your RHR. You will need a watch, timer, or clock on your phone that counts seconds.

- First thing upon rising, sit or lie down (sitting might increase RHR by up to 3 BPM)
- Find your pulse (see image below)
- Count the number of beats for 20 seconds
- Multiply this by 3 to find your RHR BPM

What the test means

Your RHR should be below 70 BPM, and ideally under 60 BPM. If your result is greater than 70, this is a good indication that you should take care of your cardiovascular system. While cardiovascular fitness (and RHR) will be improved by the exercise, nutrition, and lifestyle advice in this book, a result above 70 indicates that you may need to eventually also focus on baseline movement, breathing, and gentle conditioning in addition to strength work and body composition if that is a factor for you. This is especially true if you are already training regularly. A result of over 70 BPM in the regular trainer is a strong indication that your body composition (and hence, your nutrition and lifestyle) or your conditioning work needs improvement.

Resting heart rate values for men (beats per minute)						
Age (in years)	18-25	26-35	36-45	46-55	56-65	65+
Athlete	40-52	44-50	47-53	49-54	51-56	52-55
Excellent	56-61	55-61	57-62	58-63	57-61	56-61
Good	62-65	62-65	63-66	64-67	62-67	62-65
Above Average	66-69	66-70	67-70	68-71	68-71	66-69
Average	70-73	71-74	71-75	72-76	72-75	70-73
Below Average	74-81	75-81	76-82	77-83	76-81	74-79
Poor	82+	82+	83+	84+	82+	80+

Resting heart rate values for men. The darker-shaded blocks indicate sub-optimal results and typically suggest that your body composition, conditioning, or cardiovascular fitness requires some attention.

Waist-height ratio

Various measurements are used as indicators of overall metabolic health and later health risk. Body fat percentage, as measured by reliable tools (such as DEXA), is the 'gold standard,' but other measures, especially body mass index (BMI), are commonly used in both clinical practice and research due to their ease of use.

BMI, however, is subject to distortion due to variations in muscular body composition. For example, I am by no means 'fat' – being at the lower end of the healthy range for body fat levels, but due to being a strength athlete, my BMI (at just under 30) is 'borderline obese'.

A better measure is your waist-to-height ratio. It has been demonstrated that this measure is far more accurate than BMI for predicting health outcomes, especially for the most common health concerns, including cardiovascular disease, hypertension, and diabetes.[2-5] The suggested goal is to 'keep your waist circumference to less than half your height' to protect against cardiovascular and other diseases.[4]

How to perform the test:

- Measure your height
- Measure your waist at the 'thinnest' point
- Divide your waist measure by your height

The result should be less than 0.5.

What the test means

If your result is greater than 0.5 (i.e., your waist is more than half of your height), your health priority should be to achieve a healthy body composition and reduce body fat. If it is less than 0.5, that's great! You may be better served by focusing on another goal (based on your initial assessments).

What about blood tests?

Blood tests are an important part of evaluating one's health picture, but since the tests are interrelated and can vary significantly, it is best to have them evaluated by a qualified and registered healthcare practitioner.

However, some tests are important indicators of health that everyone should be aware of. Key among these are triglycerides (TG), cholesterol, low-density lipoprotein cholesterol (LDL), high-density lipoprotein cholesterol (HDL), and glycated haemoglobin (HbA1c). Again, if these results are outside normal reference ranges, you should first consult your doctor and a qualified, registered nutrition practitioner to help you make diet and lifestyle changes tailored to your specific needs.

Notwithstanding this, the information in this book will also help maintain health and, by extension, healthy blood markers for most people.

What are the blood tests?

Glycated haemoglobin

Glycated haemoglobin (HbA1c) is haemoglobin (the protein in red blood cells that carries oxygen) which has been 'glycated', which means that sugar in the blood has become 'stuck' to it. This provides an effective way to measure your average blood glucose and the effects of glucose (sugar) exposure in the body, as glycation is a damaging process. Think of it this way, proteins in the body that have been exposed to too much sugar get 'gunked up' and can't do their job correctly.

A higher HbA1c percentage indicates poorer blood sugar control.

Triglycerides

Triglycerides are fats (lipids) in the blood. When you eat, your body converts energy it doesn't need right away into triglycerides. These are then stored in your fat cells to be released for energy between meals.

While triglycerides are essential for health, elevated levels suggest over-fuelling and are mainly related to excessive carbohydrate intake.

Elevated triglycerides can contribute to the hardening of arteries (atherosclerosis), which increases the risk of stroke, heart attack, and heart disease and is associated with obesity, type 2 diabetes, and metabolic syndrome.

Triglycerides are one of the most important markers of health.

Cholesterol

Most people are aware that cholesterol is a key indicator of poor health, but few understand its purpose and benefits. It is a waxy, fat-like substance that provides the building blocks for cell membranes and hormones such as oestrogen and testosterone, and is vital for producing vitamin D and bile acids (which aid in the digestion of fat). While cholesterol is present in many foods and has been a target for restriction, the liver produces the cholesterol that the body requires, and dietary intake is not particularly meaningful to health.

While an extremely elevated level of cholesterol is indicative of poor diet and lifestyle choices, and therefore health, it is not an independent risk factor for poor health.

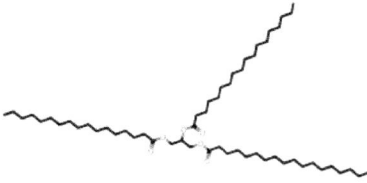

Tristearin (a Triglyceride)   Cholesterol

Because cholesterol is a lipid, it doesn't mix with blood (which is mostly water). To travel through the bloodstream, it's packaged into particles called lipoproteins. The two main types are LDL and HDL.

Low-density lipoprotein

Low-density lipoprotein (LDL) is a lipoprotein carrier that takes cholesterol from the liver to cells throughout the body. Think of it like a bus that takes passengers out to work. It is often called "bad" cholesterol because if you have too much of it in your bloodstream, it can build up on the walls of your arteries. However, it is also a critical player in the body's health.

High-density lipoprotein

High-Density Lipoprotein (HDL) is often referred to as "good" cholesterol. Using our bus analogy, this is the bus that picks up passengers after work and takes them back home; in this case, 'home' refers to the liver, where cholesterol is processed for excretion from the body.

That's why a healthy balance of LDL and HDL is essential (along with a healthy balance of all risk markers) because they work together. If one has sufficient HDL and the numbers aren't too excessive, cholesterol can be appropriately regulated without increasing the risk of atherosclerosis.

A healthy level of HDL cholesterol is protective against heart attack and stroke. It essentially helps keep your arteries clear of plaque. Higher HDL levels are desirable and indicate a lower risk of cardiovascular disease.

Other important tests for the over-40 crowd

In addition to these, liver function tests (tests of liver enzymes), ferritin, which is both a marker for iron status and inflammation, C-reactive protein, a specific measure of systemic inflammation, kidney function tests, thyroid function tests, a complete blood count, and some measures of nutritional status, might also be recommended by your doctor.

A good rule of thumb is to get a thorough checkup with blood testing annually.

Blood measure	Reference range	Optimal range
HbA1c	≤40 mmol/mol	≤40 mmol/mol
Triglycerides	<1.7 mmol/L	<1.2 mmol/L
Cholesterol	<4.0 mmol/L	Varies
LDL	<2.0 mmol/L	Varies
HDL	>1.0 mmol/L	Varies

Common nutritional tests of interest

Blood measure	Reference range	Optimal range
Vitamin D [25(OH)D]	≥50 nmol/L	100-150 nmol/L
Zinc	9-17 µmol/L	9-17 µmol/L
Folate	5-45 nmol/L	28-45 nmol/L

03

EXERCISE

Why do we exercise?

Daz: It's crazy to think that 60 years ago, my master's degree in EXERCISE physiology would have been called WORK physiology, because exercise wasn't a thing until recent history. We have a genetic instinct to conserve energy to increase our chance of survival; thus, it's no wonder exercise adherence is so low for most people.

Going much further back, however, the ancient Greeks created the first gymnasium. But besides the pursuit of physical improvement, gyms also existed for social, educational, and intellectual purposes, instilling sound morals and ethics amongst the nation's young people.

Arguably, the proper intention behind exercise has been fading ever since...

Fitness, the way it's presented to the world, is objectifying, mindless, and it has really nothing to do with moving anything, but your ego.

Carl Paoli

So, what changed? Why do we exercise for ego rather than health? Or even just for fun?

An increase in leisure time and a decrease in physically demanding lifestyles certainly have something to do with it. But if asked, most people would respond that they want to be fit and healthy. Well, in that case, we first need to define what it means to be *fit and healthy*...

"Increased capacity across broad time, modal and age domains" is a classic from CrossFit and is hard to argue with. However, what is often ignored is the 'age' part. Many people train their fitness the same way they spend their money... as if it will never run out.

Daily, high-intensity workouts, high volumes of kipping, bounding and heavy loading, all add up to aches, pains, overtraining, and eventual burnout or injury.

Exercise can become a coping mechanism to deal with the stress of daily life and work. Because we are better at adding things to our lives than taking away, we add high-intensity workouts to counteract a poor lifestyle and diet. As it becomes harder to maintain this, we blame ourselves and add even more exercise.

How can we go beyond the chasing of pain and the desire for performance to find purpose instead?

We need to discover our true why. No one is exercising ONLY to lose 5 kgs, JUST to increase the size of their biceps, or to COMPETE in an event. When we drill deeper, there is always a deeper answer.

If we discover that the motivation for exercise is more extrinsic (driven by others) than intrinsic (driven by ourselves), then we need to engage in introspection to help us find a worthy motivator. Ideally, we exercise because we CAN, not because we SHOULD.

Exercise is something that we are built to do. We are made to move and do so daily.

James Fitzgerald

To be (and remain) 'functional', we should be able to:

- Sprint
- Crawl
- Pull-up
- Push-up
- Squat
- Lunge
- Get up
- Tumble
- Carry/brace
- Strike/ brace

... and if you can't, you can rebuild that capacity!

Intensity is a thing... but not the only thing

Every strong, lean, and athletic body, from Arthur Saxon to Arnold Schwarzenegger, was built through the manipulation of the same basic training variables: load/intensity, volume, repetition range, and frequency. Exercise selection and recovery are also important variables.

When you first embark on the 'iron journey', it's remarkably simple. Try to lift more weight or complete more reps than you did the last time. Initially, that works fine! The so-called newbie gains. But at some point, progress starts to slow. Eventually, it will even begin to regress. I know that's hard to read, but unfortunately, the myth of Milo is just that, a myth. If only picking up a newborn calf and carrying it each day, and as it grew bigger and you grew stronger, eventually hauling a ton of beef around, was true!

Our genetics, training age and injury history all determine our potential. Living in the real world also means we must factor in workload, family commitments, hours of sleep, and other stressors into the mix.

The other thing about constantly adding load to the bar is that the capacity of your connective tissue and central nervous system (CNS) eventually reaches limits, increasing your risk of injury. For a normal person with real responsibilities looking to be more productive in general, testing 1RM should be low on the priority list.[6]

Cliff: Instead, one can focus on rep maxes. For example, how many reps can you do with a given weight? What load can you use in each exercise for 3, 5, or 10 reps?

Except for competitive strength athletes, no one 'needs' to test 1RM, and even for strength athletes, the frequency of maximal tests does not need to be frequent.

Interesting tests or standards that Daz has suggested are:

- A 10RM Romanian deadlift at 9 RPE
- Bulgarian split squat, 10RM with 30% of bodyweight in each hand
- 3, 5, or 10RM tests with a one-arm shoulder press (barbell, dumbbell, or kettlebell)
- Goblet squat – 50% bodyweight
- Strict pullups (RM)
- Pushups (RM)
- Kettlebell mile with 30% bodyweight in each hand
- Bodyweight (each hand) farmers carry for maximum distance
- Single-arm bench press with 30% of bodyweight (this also shows strength disparity between sides…)

Daz: If your ability to get stronger is finite, but your desire for health and function is infinite, what must change about your training?

For example, you could focus on 5+ repetition maximums rather than 1RM testing.

Reevaluate your desire to train to failure, use only central nervous system-intensive exercises, joint-unfriendly movement patterns, and your overall volume…

Failure

You don't need to train to failure to maximise your muscle size and strength. You should aim to get close on each set, but going all the way to failure is generally inferior to staying a couple of reps shy, most of the time.

Sometimes, hitting failure is useful. It guarantees a hard, stimulating set and shows you what you're capable of. It provides a reference point to track progress and determine if you're working hard enough on your other sets. However, for regular people juggling busy, stressful lives without the recovery reserves that a younger person naturally has, we're looking for the optimal training stimulus, not the maximum stimulus. Keeping 1-2 reps in the tank provides that sweet spot.

Another bonus of keeping reps in the tank is that you won't be as sore the next day. Contrary to popular belief, soreness is not a key requirement for results. If anything, excessive soreness (the type we wore as a badge of honour as 20-something-year-old strength athletes) is counter to keeping up with other sports and activities, playing with your kids, or sitting down on the toilet!

There are still ways to get a taste of pushing the limits, if you enjoy that sort of thing (like us old-school exercisers).

Periodise your efforts

E.g., Week 1: 3-4 reps in reserve, Week 2: 2-3 RIR, Week 3: 1-2 RIR, Week 4: 0-1 RIR, Week 5: 5-6 RIR (aka deload)

Push harder on peripherals

Muscles like calves, biceps, triceps and delts are all much more tolerant of sets to failure, as they create a much more localised fatigue, vs the systemic (whole body) and even CNS (nervous system) fatigue that taking bigger muscles (like the quads, hamstrings, spinal erectors etc) to failure with compound movements in a movement like 20-rep back squats.

Compound vs isolation

Similar to the last point, you may find that you can engage larger muscles closer to failure if you do so with isolation movements that, again, have a more localised than systemic effect—for example, leg extensions versus back squats for the quadriceps.

Three recent studies that support this (using trained subjects) are:

1. Carroll et al. 2019

One group failed on at least one set of every exercise, and another used relative intensity to ensure they stayed well away from failure. The study lasted 10 weeks, and the results were similar across the groups.[7]

2. Santanielo et al. 2020

This was a within-subject design, meaning the subjects trained one leg to failure and stopped short of failure on the other leg. They used leg presses and leg extensions. Quad growth and leg press 1RM increased more in the non-failure leg over 10 weeks.[8]

3. Andersen et. al. 2021

This study was similar to the above - subjects trained each leg using unilateral leg press and leg extensions over nine weeks. This time, the researchers used velocity loss to determine how close to failure to go. On one leg, they ended the sets after only a 15% velocity loss (probably with more than five reps in reserve). The other leg's sets were stopped at 30% velocity loss (probably <5 reps RIR). There were no significant differences in muscle growth between groups.[9]

The idea that the last ~5 reps before failure are "effective reps" because they involve both full motor unit recruitment and slow contraction velocities is still useful. These are important components of muscle growth. However, emerging evidence suggests that it's more nuanced than that. For us, 40+ athletes, training should feel challenging, but you don't need to push to the point of failure.

Movements for improvement, not injury

Instead of Deadlifts, try Sumo, Romanian deadlifts, Single-leg Romanian deadlifts, Trap Bar deadlifts, Jefferson curl, Hip extension, and Russian Swings. Let your own body type and what feels best during and after your sessions guide you on which movements to prioritise. Notwithstanding that, discomfort and inability to perform certain variations might also give you helpful information about what aspects of mobility or posture you may need to work on for health and longevity. For example, I (**Cliff**) find that I am strongest in a narrow stance conventional deadlift, because I have always been a 'back lifter.' When I use a very wide stance in a sumo deadlift, I inevitably strain my adductors (the muscles that pull the legs together).

However, this also gives me useful information that a) I need to work on hip mobility, and doing so really reduces the risk of back and hip pain, and b) that a squat-style deadlift, which is like a sumo-style but slightly narrower (usually in one's strongest squat position), is also a good 'middle-ground' for me.

Instead of back squat: front squat, Zercher squat/lift, goblet squat, double kettlebell or dumbbell squat, safety bar squat, belt squat, cyclist squat, split squat, lunge, step up.

Instead of squat snatch or clean: power snatch/clean, hang power snatch/clean, dumbbell snatch/clean, Russian swings.

Concepts & strategies

Movements over muscles

There's nothing wrong with training like a bodybuilder, performing lots of single-joint exercises on a complex split program. It just doesn't always give the biggest bang for your buck (in this case, your 'buck' being time). Training coordinated movement patterns has a greater crossover to daily life and is more likely to yield functional benefits in everyday activities, such as picking up a suitcase and lifting your child out of a car seat. You're also able to expose the body to greater overall loading when using big compound movements like squats and deadlifts than with isolated exercises used to target the same or similar muscle groups.

Follow a progressive approach to building strength

Progressive overload is the key concept of strength training. To put it simply, if you can lift more over time, you're getting stronger.

The example often used to illustrate this is the story of Milo, a 6th-century wrestler from Croton in *Magna Graecia* (Greek settlements in southern Italy). The legend (which may be apocryphal) claims that Milo lifted and carried a newborn calf every day, thereby strengthening himself as the calf grew into a bull.

A challenge to this approach, as we have already mentioned, is that you cannot increase the load you use every day, every week, or even every month as an advanced lifter. Sure, as a novice lifter, this is possible for weeks and months, but for every lifter, there comes a time when you hit a wall. That's why programming tactics and strategies (which we'll discuss later) are crucial to training the body to perform movements with greater loads over time.

Over time is the critical phrase because it doesn't matter so much what you lift on any given day, or whether it was more than the last session or last week. What matters is that, over the long term, with inevitable ups and downs, the weights you are using are increasing.

Leave two or more reps in the bank

There seems to be a bit of an unwritten rule that you need to train hard (which isn't wrong...) and that 'hard' means training to failure all the time... However, training to complete muscular failure increases your risk of injury and burnout. It's also not the most effective way to get stronger. Let me explain...

Being 'strong' is a function of a progressive approach to improving movement under load. Therefore, the approach we take to any other learning also applies to developing strength. For example, suppose you want to improve your jump shot in basketball. In that case, you don't go to the court, shoot progressively uglier shots (because you're becoming fatigued) until you can't lift your arms, and then wait many days until you have recovered enough to do it all over again!

If you followed this approach, you wouldn't experience enough *quality* practice to optimally improve, and more worryingly, you would be practising using poorer movement patterns. So, you wouldn't be training for your desired outcome. The better approach would be to hit the court more frequently (even multiple times per day), shoot perfectly, and call it a day whenever your focus or physical condition deteriorates.

The same methodology applies to strength development. While bodybuilders often still train to failure (although this is changing), that is because the way they look is of primary importance. It doesn't really matter whether the movement pattern is optimised. Which isn't to say that bodybuilders aren't strong (they often are), but strength athletes aim to perfect their movements under increasingly heavy loads over time. This approach maximises strength development while mitigating injury risk and reducing unnecessary muscle soreness, allowing them to spend more time practising perfectly.

How do we apply this to our training?

We should strive to execute our lifts with perfect form (which is individual). Secondly, by leaving a few reps in the bank, we can ensure that we aren't hitting the point of breakdown, which will hinder our learning of the skill (of that movement) and put us at greater risk of overreaching and burnout.

There are several ways that people quantify this in the strength world:

Repetitions in reserve (RIR)

This is the nerdy way of saying what was previously discussed. Reps in reserve means how many additional reps you think you could have completed. For example, if I performed eight repetitions in my squat and could have completed 10, that would be two repetitions in reserve, or 2RIR.

Rate of perceived exertion (RPE)

The rate of perceived exertion has slightly different definitions in the fields of strength and endurance, which can cause some confusion. In endurance training, it can serve as a way to quantify the experience of a training session. On a scale of 1 to 10, how difficult was the session? This is like a '10-point must' system in boxing and mixed martial arts.

Reps at XRM

Another way to quantify rep ranges is to perform a certain number of reps at a repetition maximum. For example, performing five repetitions at a weight that is your previous best for 10 repetitions would be five reps at 10RM.

Note: this is an excellent way to quantify starting weights in a strength cycle and many of the 'old timers' would perform rep and set schemes of around 3-5 sets of 5, beginning a cycle at a 10RM weight and increasing the load (usually by 2-5%) per week until new bests were achieved and then taking a week or two to 'deload' by either focusing on different movements (i.e., an 'easy' bodybuilding plan) or reducing the load, frequency, or volume, or taking a week off.

Finish your workout feeling fresh

Several of the great lifters of yesteryear were known for 'leaving it there.' In other words, once they hit a max, whether it be an actual personal best, a training maximum (within a cycle), or a daily max (what you feel is a comfortable maximum on any given day, dependent on how you're feeling), they would leave the training session or that lift. This concept also included designing training programs that would be challenging (in some cases, significantly so), but that would still conclude before extreme fatigue set in.

This can be especially important for the over-40 athlete, as there's no point in smashing yourself in the gym only to have no energy left for work, business, family, and pursuits of passion. Sure, there's also a place for doing the occasional *challenge workout* where you do higher-than-usual or even downright crazy volumes, loads, or density within a session. But these are once-in-a-while workouts, not your meat and potatoes. In fact, overdoing these types of workouts is likely to stall your strength gains and predispose you to a far greater risk of injury and systemic neuromuscular tension – a key cofactor in chronic pain.

A good rule of thumb for program design is that if you can achieve optimal training volume for your desired goal, your strength is increasing over time, AND you finish your workout with some energy left in the tank, you're on track for much of your training cycle.

The great strength coach Dan John describes these workouts as park bench (daily, easily repeatable workouts) vs bus bench (when you have a specific goal and need to front up, at a particular time and get shit done!).

If you hit a personal best, call it a day

As I mentioned above, generally, if you hit a personal record (PR) or personal best (PB), an excellent strategy for longevity is to 'leave it there.' The temptation is to try another PB, and sometimes you'll be able to do that; hell, sometimes maybe you even should! However, the general rule, which should only be broken rarely, is to hit a PB and then either call it a day, switch to your next exercise, or perhaps do a back-off set or two if you are feeling exceptionally strong or fresh.

Like many of the tips in this book, this was a key training tactic of many of the strength legends of yesteryear.

Do the plan

I've been guilty of wanting to 'do it all' within a training plan. The reality, though, is that you simply can't. You can't do every exercise or train for every desired outcome in each training cycle. So, set a plan and a timeframe for it (usually between three and six weeks) and stick to it for the entire time. Notwithstanding very minor fine-tuning, or when injuries or niggles might cause you to adjust the plan, as a rule, set the plan and stick to it!

Finish the plan

I'm a program-hopper by nature... When I set a new plan for myself, I hit the gym with renewed passion and energy... and then inevitably wonder if I should be doing some combination of more volume, less volume, different exercises, more or fewer exercises, ad infinitum!

If I were to constantly change the plan according to my whims (which I was guilty of at times in my younger years), I wouldn't be able to move forward consistently, nor would I be able to see what works and what doesn't. That's why, in the past, I loved training under a coach.

Nowadays, after many years of training myself, I have a firm rule: create the plan, follow the plan (see above), and complete **the plan**! Whether it's 3 weeks, 6 weeks, 12 weeks, or another duration, start the plan, do the plan, finish the plan.

This doesn't mean that you should stick blindly to a plan, though. If you are seriously stalled, get injured, have a niggle, or something else comes up that *necessitates* a change, then do it. But, let's face it, 90% of the time, the plan 'as written' is the plan that should be completed without tinkering.

Leave the psych-up music, smelling salts, pre-workouts (and chalk!) for occasional max days

A fantastic autoregulation technique for many of your training cycles is to leave all the external aids and psych-up devices and methods for the occasional workout in which you want to go 'all out.' Most of your training should be greasing the groove to improve the skill of strength, and you don't need to be jacked up on Mountain Dew to do that!

If you find that you need lifting aids, truckloads of caffeine, smelling salts, and psych-up music to get through your workout, I'd say that is either a failure of programming or an indication that your diet and lifestyle are not conducive to recovery.

Some people can train 'on the wire' most of the time, but these individuals are few and far between. I'd hazard a guess that many of them are using other *supplements* (ahem... you know what I'm sayin'...) to help them train at this excessive intensity all the time, or they are pro or semi-pro athletes with little else to do but train and recover.

Even limiting the use of chalk and straps for much of your training can be helpful, as it limits the load to what you could lift on any given day, under any circumstances. Of course, if you live in a very humid area, chalk may be necessary for safety and to support appropriate training loads.

The key takeaway is that you should be able to build strength consistently without needing to hype yourself up excessively. Developing this capacity for calm strength allows for more sustainable progress, especially for athletes and everyday individuals with other 'life stuff' on their plates.

Minimum & optimal effective training doses

Optimal and minimal effective training volumes vary significantly among individuals. Notable examples of this can be found in the fantastic book "The Purposeful Primitive" by Marty Gallagher, where he outlines the training strategies of powerlifters and bodybuilders he has coached or trained with over his many decades in the iron game. In this book, we can see that world champion strength athletes might train with short sessions only a couple of times per week (and with mostly singles and therefore, *extremely* low volume), such as Mark Chaillet, or with frequent sessions done throughout the day, akin to the squatting program of the strength legend of yesteryear, Paul Anderson.

The primary consideration of any training system is that you are (on balance) getting stronger and/or gaining muscle over time. If you're progressing, your training is both fulfilling and challenging, complementing your lifestyle and health, then it's the right plan for you. And, of course, plans and training styles can also change over time.

Having said that, the research can give us an idea of how much training volume most people need to get results. The table below outlines some ranges derived from the current research.[10,11]

Goal	Reps per set*	Sets per week	Minimum effective dose	Optimal frequency per movement/ body part
Hypertrophy (muscle gain)	6-15	12-28	4 sets per muscle group per week**	1-4+
Strength	1-6	>5-10	4 sets per muscle group per week	~4 – upper body 2-4 – lower body

Even within these minimum effective doses and optimal ranges, there is considerable flexibility. One can, and should, alter their training to suit their lifestyle, recovery ability, and desire to train.

A volume obsession is evident in the current discourse within evidence-based training circles. However, while it is true that 'volume is king' for hypertrophy, this also lacks nuance, and three points provide essential context to the research findings.

Training volume is individual-dependent

Everyone has a unique ability to recover, which is dependent in turn on their physiology and, more importantly, their psychosocial milieu (work, stress, family, nutrition, sleep, and environment).

There is wide inter-individual variability

Some people excel with low volumes of training. People like Mark Chaillet, who won world titles in powerlifting training just two days per week and simply working up to a max single of bench and squat on one day, and deadlifts on the other, or Dorian Yates, who won six consecutive Mr Olympia titles using 1-2 working sets to failure and using far lower volumes than most other bodybuilders of his era.

Volume is important – but returns are diminishing

More is often helpful, especially for gaining muscle (although it is less so for strength), but the benefits of increasing training volume diminish the more you add. This can be critical to an individual because they might experience diminishing or even negative returns from increased volume much earlier than others. This is due to their recovery being hampered by poorer sleep, high stress, suboptimal nutrition, or physical factors such as chronic health conditions.

Even as little as one set per week is still effective for strength and muscle gains. In fact, while there is a linear trend for muscle mass increases associated with higher volumes, the clustering of studies with lower-than-optimal volumes suggests that the difference between lower and higher volumes is only slightly meaningful. See, for example, the greatest magnitude of effect and clustering in ~3-10 sets per week in this recent meta-regression by Pelland et al.[12]

Volume & Hypertrophy: **Volume & Strength:**

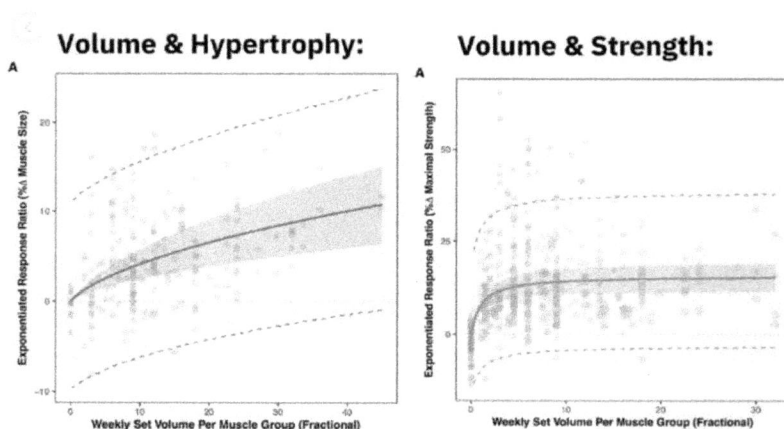

Prioritise strength training

Daz: I talk with my clients a lot about the importance of strength work, and there are many reasons for this:

- Increased strength will potentially have the most significant impact on the quality of life for the average person.
- Increased muscle mass will mean less body fat due to increased metabolism.
- Improved posture and prevention of injury-related falls in older age.

- Translation to sport performance.
- Translation to everyday life tasks - changing a car tyre, lifting kids, carrying groceries, climbing stairs, etc.
- Strength-based movements typically require the most practice, both because they can be technical to learn and to maximise safety. Thus, programming them more often is crucial.
- It's also the type of fitness training that continues to offer opportunities to get better and for learning. Decades into a fitness practice, and you'll still be working on some aspect of strength development, whereas aerobic capacity tends to have gone as far as it's going to.
- Spending the entire workout, and then multiple workouts per week on high-intensity conditioning, leads to overuse issues on joints, cumulative fatigue, and potentially over-training, not to mention being ineffective for long-term health and fitness goals.

Far too many fitness programs don't prioritise strength, including some of the most popular ones, and they certainly wouldn't dream of devoting entire workouts to strength and accessory movements. The perception exists, from both the practitioner and the provider, that fitness is only fun if it's fast and furious. Intuitively, it makes sense: the more you move, the more you sweat, and the more you sweat, the more you burn, right?! (Nope...)

Intensity

One aspect of fitness for the general population changed irrevocably with the advent of CrossFit. Everyone who trains in a functional fitness gym loves an intense workout.

But what about the workouts that aren't so intense?

It's pretty instinctive to feel like heart rate, heavy breathing, and fatigue are the only indicators of effective training, but that's not how the body works.

The best way to 'tone,' to lose body fat, to get leaner, to get a six pack, to build a resilient, injury-proof, and healthy body, is by building muscle (and strength). The most effective way to achieve this is through strength training, rather than cardio, interval training, or metabolic conditioning (also known as metcons). If you only work at high intensity, you will eventually break. It may be physical, resulting from an injury or overtraining, or it may be mental, as often seen when people suddenly say, "I've had enough!"

The body/mind can only take so much intensity. None of this is meant to diminish the importance of higher-intensity interval training, met-cons, or cardio, as they all have a valuable place in a well-rounded exercise routine. It is simply to point out the 'biggest bang for your buck' from training for health and longevity.

Deep practice

We love a bit of mindfulness! There is immense value in slowing down and experiencing every aspect and every second of each rep, both self-assessing what is moving where and how it feels, and simply enjoying the sensation of what your body can do. As we progress in our health and fitness journey, developing a more patient approach is the only way to reach the finish line... which, of course, is the last day on this earth. Strength training is a test of pure patience; learn to love it and you'll win life's race.

Things I would tell myself as a young lifter

Cliff: Back in the day, competing in All-Round lifting, I did OK. I won a few comps, set a couple of records, and performed feats of strength at expos and on TV. But looking back, I never truly became strong. It wasn't even so apparent 'back in the day' as strength sports were yet to undergo their recent renaissance, driven in no small part by the increasing popularity of CrossFit and other 'functional' training brands that have inevitably led to people being exposed to Powerlifting and Olympic Lifting and eventually crossing over to these sports.

Case in point, several of our recent Commonwealth Games Olympic lifters are high-level CrossFitters, first exposed to Olympic lifting in that sport.

Now, looking back, I can see that I was lucky that there weren't as many people competing in strength sports back in the day. This is not to say that I am deriding my achievements. I'm proud of the records I set and those I surpassed in unofficial exhibitions. It's just that I could have been so much more as a strength athlete with that inevitable and always unattainable (in-the-moment) benefit of hindsight.

So, with that in mind, here's what I would tell 'me' in my twenties:

Don't rush

As a young lifter, I wanted to emulate my buddy, the late, great Steve Angell and be regarded as one of the strongest dudes on the planet! The problem was that I was always focused on the records and titles, rather than training properly to achieve longevity in the sport. Consequently, I allowed too many maximum attempts and attempted a far too steep progression strategy for my lifting. While I did hit decent numbers, they were nowhere near what they could have been if I had taken more time to *create a wider base.*

Create a wider base

You can build a taller structure if it has a wider base. The same is true for training, but people (my previous self included) don't want to spend long months working with sub-maximal weights, maintaining perfect form, and focusing on their weak points. But working on these weak points, and it should be said, working on the BIG lifts that maximally improve strength overall, and continuing to build overall tolerance to strength training, are critical to developing sustainable, long-term strength. You might even surprise yourself at how strong you can become!

Work your weak points

I tended to perform vanity lifts that I knew I was strong at. It's fair to say I was a bit of a 'back and grip' lifter, putting up decent numbers in one-hand deadlifts, rack lifts, and other grip and muscle lifts. The thing is, I hadn't built the foundation to be putting up those numbers at my body weight. Particularly, I should have focused more on gaining prodigious levels of leg strength.

As I've discussed recently with Daz, I believe that leg strength is equally important for someone who tends to be a hinge/back lifter as it is for someone who is a 'leg lifter' (think of the difference between a hinge-style deadlift and sumo or squat-style deadlift). Having the foundation of support that incredible leg strength and drive provide helps retain greater stability, hip position, and reduces the risk of injury for the hinge lifter.

Most of us should incorporate more squats and lunges into our workouts.

Squat more!

Carrying on from the point above, my legs were far weaker than my back. While I have squatted some decent poundage (180 kg for a triple at a bodyweight of 75 kg), these were aberrations achieved after dedicated squat blocks. Much of my training failed to incorporate enough volume, technique work, and intention on good ol' squatting. When I focused on it, I aimed to get some decent numbers up, rather than following better strategies like not rushing, concentrating on a foundation of lower-body strength, and training sub-maximally (i.e., *don't fail*).

Don't fail

I had my best strength increases training as an Olympic lifter (although I was using it to train for All-Round) under the tutelage of the great New Zealand Olympic Weightlifting team coach

Richard Dryden and Commonwealth Games medallist Nigel Avery.

Sure, a big part of this was because, before this, my Olympic lifting technique was rubbish! However, it was also due to the progressive, sub-maximal, high-frequency approach inherent in Olympic Weightlifting. A significant part of that training style involved building a base, avoiding rushing, maintaining a very low frequency of reaching true maximums, and performing a large volume of squats.

I failed far too much in my lifting outside of my time in Olympic lifting, and this led to not just sub-optimal results but also predisposed me to the severe back injuries that subsequently put me out of competition for many years. I also didn't have the physical structure to be the best lifter I could be, and so, *I needed to get bigger.*

Get bigger

I lifted in the under-75 kg category. I'm 5'9" and this is just too small. I was, by far, one of the most linear athletes competing in that class, and I believe the lack of mass not only affected my strength but also reduced my structural stability under load.

I also actively tried to stay very lean and was constantly fighting an internal struggle between gaining muscle, losing fat, and preserving optimal energy levels to support hormonal balance, offset the risk of overtraining, and ensure adequate rest, sleep, stress modulation, and overall recovery.

In retrospect, I can now see that I failed in that regard. The younger I was, the less it impacted me. Still, as I moved through my late 20s and early 30s, I experienced shorter sleeping cycles, severe muscle twitches, fatigue, lacklustre performances, and a slew of injuries; all common outcomes of chronic underfuelling.

I was ripped (and looked great for the beach), but I felt like I was on an energy and mood roller-coaster most of the time. This serves as a great reminder that the way we look is not always the best indicator of our overall health.

Summary

- Slow down.
- Take your time.
- Don't train to failure except for the very occasional test of your max, but make those max tests 'easy maxes.'
- Leave the gym feeling fresh.
- Eat to fuel the work required and the results desired.
- Fill out your structure.
- Set a wide foundation of strength and focus on building incredible (and lasting) leg drive and strength.

These things will set you up for a lifetime of strength and health.

Now, at 46 years of age, I am 15 kg heavier than my former competition weight (and believe me, I won't be cutting for comps!). I eat a truckload more, I'm a little fatter (though not by any means 'fat') and as a result, a heck of a lot happier. I also have a feeling that I'll become stronger, and more sustainably so, as I enter my next phase of lifting as an advanced master's lifter.

Training structure

Cliff: Most of my training involves the structure outlined in the table below. The first exercise grouping is dynamic lifts. Since various iterations of the Clean & Press/Jerk and Snatch are typically featured in major All-Round Weightlifting competitions, I dedicate a significant amount of practice time to these lifts when competing.

Notice I said 'practice.' These lifts are performed first in the session due to their complexity (you don't want to be excessively fatigued if you want to train a complex/fast lift optimally), and they function as both a warm-up for the heavy lifts to come and as light pulls to train that movement pattern

If you are fatigued (either chronically or on any given day), dynamic training (and intense conditioning work) can be counter-productive to recovery. In contrast, heavy, low-volume, compound 'grind' strength work, such as squats, deadlifts, and overhead presses, is fairly 'tonic' for the nervous system.

Next up are the 'core' strength lifts, usually based around the powerlifting trio of squats, bench press (and/or overhead pressing) and deadlifts or pulls (and all the varieties of these lifts!).

Finally, assistance work can be done at the end of the session based on the relative needs of the training cycle. For example, if you are in a body-composition (fat-loss) or conditioning-heavy phase, you might add Tabata intervals of push-ups alternated with kettlebell swings. If you are in a mass-gaining phase, you might add additional pressing and rowing variations along with heavy curls to satisfy your yearning for bigger biceps.

Exercise type	Example
Dynamic lifts	Snatch, Power Snatch Clean, Power Clean, Power Clean and Press/Jerk
'Core' strength lifts	Front Squat Military Press Bench Press Rows Deadlifts
Assistance (depending on current focus)	Conditioning (i.e., high-rep swings; pushups; weighted Tabatas or other interval training strategy; circuits or PHA training; longer distance, slower cardio) Rehab and prehab work Bodybuilding

Remember that the key element of training is the STRENGTH work. If you are short on time, tired, or exhausted, this is the component of your program you should prioritise, allowing you to drop the other elements temporarily.

If you are exhausted, it could also indicate that other aspects of your overall health regimen aren't on point. You might benefit from a deload, an active-recovery week, or a complete rest from training for up to two weeks.

To split or not to split?

Split or don't... it doesn't really matter too much, *so long as you are achieving your goals, and you are recovering well.* I tend towards whole body workouts for several reasons:

1. Most competitive lifts involve the whole body
2. It is typically preferable to train 'movements, not muscles'
3. On balance, the evidence favours (albeit slightly) a greater frequency of movements for the development of strength when volume is equated
4. It is easier for people to achieve the requisite volume for strength and muscle development by using large, complex movements more frequently, as compared to having to do a LOT of single-joint exercises in a session on a complex split program

However, there are times when I split the body up more, especially when I am not recovering well and when I feel a bit more 'banged up.' For example, I have recently been strength training twice a week (in addition to two Brazilian Jiu Jitsu sessions and two mobility sessions), focusing on a mostly lower-to-upper split. This means that I am only training each movement/muscle once per week. This might run counter to what some suggest is 'optimal' and even to what Daz and I have been saying in this book. But the rationale is that sometimes my recovery is not ideal due to work, sport (grappling), and family commitments. At these times, I often reduce the volume and frequency of training, and my results are better as a result.

How often you train and whether you should split your body (and how much) is frequently best determined by considering how long you need to recover (per muscle group) between sessions.

Estimating your recovery requirements

Here is a practical framework to help you estimate your recovery needs.

Step 1: Start with a baseline

For a challenging, heavy strength training session targeting a specific muscle group, begin with a baseline recovery window.

Baseline recovery time: 48 Hours

This is the standard, scientifically supported timeframe for muscle protein synthesis to peak and return to near-normal levels after a strenuous workout in a healthy, active individual.

Step 2: Adjust for your workout

Next, modify the baseline based on the specifics of your training session. The nature of your workouts is the most significant factor influencing recovery.

Training intensity & volume:

- **Moderate intensity/volume:** (e.g., you generally finish your sets feeling like you could have done 2-3 more reps) -> **No change**. Stay at 48 hours.
- **High intensity/high volume:** (e.g., you train to failure on multiple sets, often lift >85% of your one-rep max, or do a high number of sets) -> **Add 24 hours**.
- **Low intensity/deload:** (e.g., you are doing light technique work, or a planned deload week) -> **Subtract 24 hours**.

Muscle Group Size:

- **Small muscle groups:** (e.g., biceps, triceps, calves, shoulders) -> **Subtract 12 hours**.
- **Large muscle groups:** (e.g., quads, hamstrings, glutes, back) -> **Add 12 hours**. These larger muscles undergo more breakdown and require more resources to repair.

Type of Exercise:

- **High eccentric focus:** (e.g., movements emphasise the lowering phase, like slow negatives or Romanian deadlifts)

-> **Add 12 hours**. Eccentric contractions are known to cause more muscle damage.

Step 3: Adjust for physical & lifestyle factors

Finally, fine-tune your estimate based on your personal biology and daily habits. These factors determine the quality and speed of your body's repair processes.

Sleep Quality:

- **Poor sleep (<7 hours or interrupted): -> Add 24 hours.** This is the most critical recovery factor. Without adequate sleep, your body's repair hormones are blunted.
- **Optimal sleep (7-9 hours): -> No Change.**

Nutrition:

- **Sub-optimal nutrition:** (e.g., you are in a significant calorie deficit for fat loss, or you don't commonly meet optimal protein targets, essential fats, or you are not consuming enough vegetables, berries, and otherwise meeting micronutrient requirements) -> **Add 12 hours.** Your body lacks the immediate fuel and building blocks for repair.
- **Optimal nutrition:** (e.g., adequate calories and protein intake) -> **No Change.**

Age:

- **Ages 40+: This is us!** -> **Add 12 hours.** While training experience helps, physiological aging can naturally slow down recovery processes. Younger lifters may not need this adjustment.

Stress levels:

- **High life stress (work, personal):** -> **Add 12 hours.** Elevated levels of stress can actively hinder muscle repair.

Round up (and be pragmatic):

The estimates above are intended to allow for optimal muscle recovery, so you should round up your estimation to ensure a full recovery. If, for example, your recovery estimate worked out to 5.5 or 6 days, the best strategy would be to train each muscle group or movement pattern just once a week.

Putting It All Together: Two Examples

Example 1: The Young, Focused Lifter

A 22-year-old student performs a high-intensity arm workout (biceps and triceps). He gets 8 hours of sleep, and his nutrition is on point.

- **Baseline:** 48 hours
- **Workout Adjustment:** High Intensity (+24 hours), Small Muscle Group (-12 hours)
- **Lifestyle Adjustment:** Optimal sleep and nutrition (+0 hours)
- **Estimated Recovery Time:** 48 + 24 - 12 + 0 = **60 Hours** (or ~2.5 days, rounded up to 3 days)

Example splits:

- Full body on Monday and Thursday
- Upper-Lower split on Monday, Tuesday, Thursday, and Friday

Example 2: The Busy, Experienced Parent.

A 46-year-old with years of training experience has a very heavy leg day. She is stressed from work, has only slept 6 hours, and is in a calorie deficit to lose weight.

- **Baseline:** 48 hours
- **Workout Adjustment:** High Intensity (+24 hours), Large Muscle Group (+12 hours)
- **Lifestyle Adjustment:** Poor Sleep (+24 hours), Sub-optimal Nutrition (+12 hours), Age 40+ (+12 hours), High Stress (+12 hours)
- **Estimated Recovery Time:** 48 + 24 + 12 + 24 + 12 + 12 + 12 = **144 Hours** (or 6 days)

Example splits:

- Upper-Lower split on Monday and Tuesday (one movement/muscle per week). This type of split can work well if the person also competes in another sport.
- 'Bro Splits' training each muscle/movement once a week

This starkly different result highlights why a "one-size-fits-all" approach is ineffective. For this individual, training legs again in two or three days would be counterproductive, leading to inferior performance and an increased risk of injury.

By using this framework, you can objectively assess your recovery needs and learn to listen to the body's signals (like persistent soreness, low energy, and decreased strength) to make smarter training decisions.

Caveats to recovery estimates

The recovery estimates above are just that, estimates. Some people may want or need to train more frequently, although few would want to train less frequently than the estimates above provide. It's also important to remember that if one is on a highly periodised program that includes lighter sessions, recovery days (or weeks) or an incremental increase in volume and intensity (like programs used in Olympic and All-Round Weightlifting), one may train each movement more frequently. In fact, for strength sports, it can be preferable to train movements more frequently, while closely monitoring relative volume, intensity, and recovery ability to improve the execution of those specific movements.

Balance in training

A concept that is worth emphasising is that of 'balance' in your strength training. By this, I mean that you want to use appropriate volumes to avoid prioritising one group of muscles over another, especially an opposing muscle complex, which could precipitate postural issues and injuries.

For example, many people love to press, especially horizontal plan pressing like the Bench Press. But an over-focus on that lift, without concurrently training the 'pulling' muscles that retract and fix the scapula in position and preserve proper shoulder joint positioning, can result in shoulder injuries, pain, and ultimately are not what most of us would desire for aesthetics either – namely the rounded shoulder positioning that tightness and imbalance of those shoulder girdle muscles can lead to.

There are exceptions to this 'rule', and I know lifters who do little work for retraction, and they have BIG bench presses and healthy shoulders, but they are few and far between. Most of us would benefit from at least a 1:1 ratio of pulling to pushing exercises (and volume), and many would be even better off with a 1.5:1 or 2:1 ratio.

Similarly, many people have 'anterior dominant' lower body muscle complexes and tend to have weaker glutes and hamstrings compared to their quads, and so, focusing on hip extension (e.g., hip hinge exercises like Deadlifts, Swings, Hip Thrusts, Glute Bridges, etc.) can help to prevent imbalances in the lower body.

Do you need to periodise?

Periodisation of training is helpful because it allows one to focus on different outcomes (i.e., hypertrophy, strength, power, etc.) in distinct phases of training. However, rigid 'classic' periodisation models are unnecessary for the average gymgoer, recreational athlete, or someone who wants to be awesome. In fact, I believe that even for many athletes, these types of periodisation models don't work as well as expected.

There are many ways to skin a cat, and rigidly defined periodisation is not the only, nor the most effective way to train. To put it simply, as an over-40 athlete, the most important thing is to stick with a plan for a minimum timeframe to see results (usually longer than three weeks). After a training plan, you can refocus on what your 'next' goal is and either stick with the same or very similar plan for another cycle, adjust the plan, or start a new plan according to what is going to meet your needs best and what will challenge you and keep things fresh, motivating, and engaging.

What about deloads?

Similarly, rigid deloads performed every 3-6 weeks are often unnecessary. I'm not implying that you don't need downtime or lighter sessions or weeks; deloads work incredibly effectively for many people. However, there are many ways to approach training.

I think back to my days lifting under the tutelage of the great Olympic Weightlifting coach Richard Dryden. We never 'deloaded' per se. Instead, we would have the occasional break from training due to life's demands (such as going away for summer break) or after a major meet.

After returning, training would 'ramp up' over a cycle (typically 12 or more weeks) from relatively easy to a peak of intensity towards the end of the training phase. So, there were implicit 'deloads', but they were pretty different to the standard and US powerlifting-biased idea of a light week at the conclusion of a short training block.

Many great lifters never deload and instead take the odd break from training, usually due to other life demands (as mentioned above) rather than because it is planned within a training macrocyle and/or they autoregulate training based on how they feel on any given day or week, which in turn is based off how their life and recovery are going at that time. And the greats of the iron game would often throw in a 'pump and pose' bodybuilding-style block for a few weeks after a meet or when getting back into training to give the body a break from the repetitive strain of heavy, competition-style lifting.

In many ways, this is a far more intuitive and beneficial approach to training, especially for those with variable demands on their time and energy from life, business, and family, among other commitments.

So, deload or don't, it doesn't matter too much. Just make sure that you recognise your recovery and daily readiness within your training and take the occasional break from it.

How long can you take a break?

If you're letting *life* determine, at least in part, when you're going to deload by engaging in different activities or taking a complete break from training, the question inevitably arises: *Just how long can I take a break without affecting my progress?*

Research suggests that taking up to 3 weeks off has little effect on strength,[13] so, you shouldn't worry about one or two training holidays per year. Of course, suffice it to say that you must earn your rest!

If you train for one week, take three weeks off, and then repeat the cycle shortly after, you will experience detraining.

04

CARDIO

Cardiovascular training, or aerobic exercise, similarly to our recent volume obsession, is touted as a 'must-do' by experts. However, I think that in the 'hierarchy of needs' of training, specific cardiovascular training, and even other forms of crossover exercise like high-intensity interval training (HIIT), anti-glycolytic training, and 'metabolic conditioning', provide less of a bang-for-buck than strength training and residual activity like just getting in your 7000+ steps per day anyway you can.

It's also fair to say, despite what many 'experts' spout on social media, that strength training provides cardiovascular benefits, and possibly sufficient cardiovascular benefits to offset later health and mortality risks.

None of which is to say that you *shouldn't* perform cardio; in fact, you should!

But, more importantly, you shouldn't prioritise cardio training over strength work unless, of course, you have a passion for endurance AND you are still getting a minimum effective dose of strength training every week.

HIIT, AGT, etc.

Steady State (e.g., Zone 2) Cardio

Residual Activity

Strength Training

So, the question remains: Should you do cardio, and if so, how and when?

The answer, despite what you may think after reading the previous paragraphs, is a resounding yes! However, I don't believe that one should stress too much about the type or volume of cardio training, especially if they are still integrating the general habit of exercise and prioritising strength training.

I (Cliff) tend to get 7000+ steps per day from running around after kids and doing housework (although I'm sure Bella gets a lot more steps than I do!). So, I focus on participating in my sport (Brazilian

Jiu Jitsu), which provides a lot of crossover to cardiovascular fitness, and then either incorporate some light (Zone 2) style cardio at a minimum effective dose of around 90 minutes per week, usually by getting in a 15-minute session after my morning strength training or before lunch. I also add an anti-glycolytic or HIIT circuit to my routine on 1-2 days of the week following strength training.

Cardio definitions

When I'm working with clients, I find that a lot of them are confused by the terminology used in training in general, and in cardiovascular training in particular. Some of the terms I have used in this chapter are:

Zone 2 cardio

Zone 2 is low-intensity, steady-state exercise performed at the highest level of intensity one can while still burning predominantly fat as a fuel. Many argue that it is the most important type of exercise for overall health, endurance, and longevity, although I believe that strength training trumps even Zone 2!

In Zone 2, the muscles are working hard enough to stimulate adaptations of the cardiovascular system and increase both the number and efficiency of mitochondria, enabling the body to use more fat at higher intensities of exercise (metabolic flexibility).

The easiest and most practical way to ensure you are in Zone 2 is the **Talk Test.** Simply put, you can comfortably hold a conversation while exercising. If you could sing a song, the intensity is too low, and if you are gasping for breath, the intensity (specifically for Zone 2 exercise) is too high.

A nice aspect of Zone 2 cardio is that it doesn't really tax your recovery systems, making it a great addition (not an alternative) to your strength training, which can also facilitate recovery.

- **Minimum effective dose:** Around 90 minutes per week
- **Optimal dose:** 150+ minutes per week

Anti-glycolytic training

Anti-glycolytic training (AGT) is a method of conditioning that focuses on performing repeated bursts of explosive, high-power work while actively avoiding the metabolic fatigue associated with the glycolytic (sugar-burning) energy system.

The goal is to train the **ATP-PC (phosphocreatine) system**, which provides immediate energy for efforts lasting about 10-15 seconds. This is achieved by using a specific work-to-rest ratio:

- **Work:** Very short, explosive bursts of effort (e.g., 10-15 seconds).

- **Rest:** Long and complete rest periods (e.g., 45-90 seconds). This long rest allows the aerobic system to fully replenish the phosphocreatine stores in the muscles, enabling the next set to be performed with the same high level of power and quality, without accumulating the metabolic byproducts (like lactate) that cause the "burn."

In short, it is training for power and efficiency without the metabolic stress.

High-intensity interval training

HIIT training involves repeated bouts of maximal or near-maximal effort followed by short periods of rest or low-intensity active recovery.

The goal of HIIT is to intentionally overload the glycolytic energy system and push the body into a significant oxygen debt. The work intervals are performed at an intensity that is unsustainable for more than a short period (e.g., 20-60 seconds), and the rest periods are deliberately incomplete.

- **Work:** Short to moderate intervals of "all-out" effort (e.g., 20-60 seconds).
- **Rest:** Short, incomplete rest periods that are not long enough for full recovery.

This creates a massive metabolic disturbance, leading to the "burn" and breathlessness. The primary adaptations from HIIT come from the body learning to tolerate and buffer the metabolic byproducts and the powerful "afterburn" effect, known as EPOC (Excess Post-exercise Oxygen Consumption).

In short, it is training for metabolic conditioning and tolerance of high-intensity fatigue.

HIIT training requires more recovery reserve than either low-volume strength training, Zone 2 cardio, or AGT.

This table summarises the key differences between HIIT and AGT:

Feature	AGT	HIIT
Primary goal	Develop explosive power and work capacity without fatigue.	Improve metabolic conditioning and fatigue tolerance.
Energy system	ATP-PC (anaerobic, alactic)	Glycolytic (anaerobic, lactic)
Work interval	Short & explosive (10-15 seconds)	Short to moderate & "all-out" (20-60 seconds)
Rest interval	Long & complete (45-90 seconds)	Short & incomplete (10-60 seconds)
Feeling/sensation	Fresh, powerful, and repeatable. No "burn."	Breathless, high heart rate, significant muscle "burn."
Primary adaptation	Improved power output and faster recovery between efforts.	Increased $\dot{V}O_2$ max and improved tolerance for metabolic stress.

05

MOBILITY

Cliff: 'Mobility' is critical to health and performance, and yet, it's commonly misunderstood. As compared to flexibility, which is the ability to move a limb through a (larger) range of motion, mobility refers to functional ability (especially strength) through an optimised range of motion. Rather than just being more 'bendy,' this involves having the strength, muscle recruitment, activation, and postural stability needed to move joints through ranges of motion that are conducive to safe performance.

Do you need to do mobility training?

Ultimately, the answer is a qualified no, as full-range strength training improves range of motion as much as stretching.[14] However, mobility work done in addition to strength training, either before and/or intermittently, is beneficial, predominantly because we 'pattern' ourselves into specific postures within our modern lifestyle.

We are generally more sedentary and move in far fewer integrated movement patterns and plans than we have evolved to. Additionally, the effects of stress and less-than-optimal nutrition on muscular tension and pain further contribute to poorer posture, activation, and mobility. Therefore, due to the volume of 'anti-mobility' lifestyle factors, most of us will benefit from incorporating more mobility work into our training regimen and daily routine.

It's also important to remember that as we get older, we typically move less overall, as we are less likely to be out running around in random pickup games of touch and basketball. Our recovery ability is not as good as it was when we were younger.

What does this have to do with mobility?

Even though full-range weightlifting and other activities are as beneficial as stretching and mobility, if we are doing less of these and potentially engaging in more 'anti-postural' activities, adding mobility work (which requires little in the way of recovery) helps to redress this deficit in 'mobilising' activities.

Having said all of that, most of my mobility work comes in the form of full-range All-Round and Olympic-style lifting. My pre-workout regimen typically involves performing sets of the exercises I intend to do with lighter weights, along with a lot of auto-cueing and intention to activate and mobilise. Of late, I have made an effort to add 5-10 minutes of extra mobility work in the morning (outside... more on that later) to complement this.

I also perform mobility exercises throughout the day, primarily focusing on various sitting postures, bodyweight squat sits, arm swings, pike arches (also known as up-down dog), and 'perfect stretches.' My favourite daily corrective exercise, especially when I'm sitting a lot at work, is the 'static postural lunge.' This reactivates the glutes, which have been deactivated by prolonged periods of sitting, and provides an active stretch through functional movement and range of motion for the hip flexors, including the oft-neglected rectus femoris (the 'long' quadriceps muscle that crosses both the hip and knee joints). And for the neck, back, and shoulder girdle, I add band face pulls and pull-aparts (I keep a band and a foam roller in my office).

Daz, however, is far more well-versed in mobility... Over to you, mate!

Daz: Ask almost anyone what they want to achieve from their workout routine, and you'll hear fat loss or muscle gain, or 'tone up' or 'be a bit fitter...'

What you'll rarely hear as a top priority is to be more mobile. However, in the long term, your ability to get into a squat and put your arms above your head will count far more towards your quality of life than how much extra weight you can hoist through those positions.

I often use the example of an ex-All Black, walking into my gym in his 50s, with a handful of joint surgeries, metal pins, bone spurs, and worn-out cartilage to deal with. At his peak, he could back squat 180 kg and was one of the fastest players in the world.

What do you think was more important to him now? To vainly chase after his old squat PR? To get his 100m dash time down again? Is it about being able to get down to the floor without pain to play with his grandchildren?

In this chapter of life, he was much better served with Turkish Get-ups and Bear Crawls than heavy Squats and gruelling circuits.

Yes, strength and speed are still necessary, but as we've mentioned often in this book, we're looking for the optimum, not the maximum. Chasing maximums always comes with a cost. Just ask the bionic man referenced above.

So, what is mobility exactly?

There are two important terms to define...

1. **Flexibility:** the range of motion that can be PASSIVELY displayed at a joint (e.g. reaching forward and touching your toes with straight legs).

2. **Mobility:** the range of motion that can be ACTIVELY displayed at a joint (e.g., a straight-legged high kick in front of the body).

Your passive range of motion will exceed your active range, i.e., if I were to lift your foot at the apex of your high kick, you would get higher than you could on your own.

This is your nervous system protecting your joints and muscles from harm by imposing a kind of 'limiter.' You need to be able to control (stabilise) your limbs at whatever range you can move them to. If the difference between your active and passive ranges is significant, you have a decreased ability to control that joint actively. So, while being flexible is a good thing, being mobile is even better.

Think of it as a formula:

Mobility = flexibility + stability

We want to be able to both move our joints through their full range of motion and also control them. Picture action movie star Jean Claude van Damme doing the splits on two chairs. That is flexibility (full range of motion at the hips), but also stability (the strength to support his bodyweight on the chairs with the hip musculature)

Most people are acutely aware of their mobility (or lack thereof), but the traditional methods used to improve it are often inefficient and tedious. The length of the muscle is usually perceived as the limiting factor. Thus, long, static-stretching sessions are commonly prescribed for improvement. While static stretching can increase flexibility, it does a poor job of addressing neurological limitations and makes little to no improvement in stability. It's still beneficial; it can serve as a useful cooldown practice after a workout, helping to upregulate the parasympathetic nervous system, which is essential for relaxation and recovery.

But as a bang-for-buck method, improving your mobility will have the greatest carryover to your workout preparation, performance, and safety.

Types of mobility training

Joint rotations

Start with the neck; up and down, side to side, ear to shoulder, each side, and then some slow rotations, then a few forward and backward to reset your 'text neck.'

Next, the shoulders, up and down shrugs, then move the shoulder blades forward and back, then try inwards and outwards, imagining them 'sliding' over your rib cage. Then take a straight arm and rotate your shoulder through full circles, in both directions.

Then, the elbows, wrists, fingers, and continue down the body, including the hips, knees, feet, and toes.

Taking five minutes in the morning to move all your joints through their full passive ranges of motion won't seem like much at the time, but add that up over 10 years of real-world wear and tear on your body, and you've mitigated it with over 300 hours of mobility work!

Movement flows

This is a favourite of mine, because it's a great way to tick lots of boxes in a short amount of time. They are athletic and graceful, focused and mindful. They can be performed in a small space with no equipment needed, and, of course, they drastically improve your mobility. Check out AnimalFlow.com for some interesting applications of movement flow.

Dynamic stretching

Good old-fashioned, 'getting ready to run a race' drills. Arm and leg swings, high-knee skips, butt-kickers, side shuffles, backpedals, and walking lunges all take your joints and muscles through an extensive range of motion, with extra load applied either from the weight of your body or a little speed on the limbs.

Loaded stretching

This form of mobility work is currently immensely popular. It can include simple modifications to traditional strength exercises to add increased stretch to the end range (which may also improve hypertrophy), or entire schools of thought based around it, such as FRS (Functional Range Systems).

You'll see examples of exercises that incorporate loaded stretching in some of the workouts included in this book.

Sample mobility tests

- Sumo Good Morning (hip flexion and abduction)
- Wall Squat (shoulder flexion, thoracic extension, hip, and ankle flexion)
- Crab Walk (hip extension, shoulder, and wrist extension)
- Seiza Squat and Sit (hip, knee, ankle, and toe flexion)
- Turkish Get Up (hip extension, shoulder abduction)

06

WEAK POINTS & POSTURAL ISSUES

Several common strength, positional, or postural issues are encountered by people as they age. These are especially relevant for the AA40 athlete.

The most common of these are:

- Tight and weak hip flexors
- Weak or overused quadratus lumborum
- Excessive kyphosis/lordosis
- Forward head carriage
- Poor shoulder carriage
- Lower arm flexion/extension imbalances
- Poor bracing (anti-movement) control of the core

Corrective Rx for common issues

As we age, most of us experience aches, niggles, and shoulder injuries. A combination of sedentary lifestyles, poor training practices, and work-related overuse injuries can all lead us to shoulder, hip, back and neck pain.

Thankfully, we can alleviate a lot of this pain and dysfunction through a combination of preventative exercise, diet and lifestyle.

Tight and weak hip flexors

Years ago, we were commonly taught that, due to our modern lifestyle, which involves limited activity and a lot of sitting, our hip flexors (especially the Psoas muscle) become 'dominant' in comparison to the hip extensors (the hamstrings and glutes). However, this is seldom seen in practice. More often, we see that people have tight and *weak* hip flexors. Therefore, the exercise prescription to ensure better hip position (and consequently, better back health) can't just involve excessive stretching of the psoas without also strengthening the hip-flexor complex and the hip extensors.

Hip mobility drills

Strengthening the hip flexors

Many people claim that the hip flexors should not be trained directly. There is some truth to that, but at the same time, you shouldn't fear involving your hip flexors in strength movements!

In fact, you ***should*** strengthen the hip flexors. The best way to achieve this is by incorporating enhanced cueing during your squats and occasionally doing some hanging leg raises.

Usually, people either 'drop' into a squat or resist the movement down. However, to actively engage your hip flexors when squatting, imagine *pulling* yourself down into the squat. Imagine that there is resistance trying to pull you up and actively pull yourself down by hinging back and pulling yourself down *between* your legs. If you're having trouble feeling this, mimic the movement with a partner by lying on the ground (hold on to something) and have your partner hold your feet. Now, as if you are squatting down, pull them towards you using your hip flexors. You can also do this with a band offering resistance against the eccentric or downward phase of a bodyweight squat.

Leg raises are a great integrative exercise for the entire body, specifically targeting the hip flexors. The reason I like these is that they are a 'functional' movement that crosses over to human survival skills. For example, imagine you fall off something and manage to catch onto something. Great, you've survived.... for the moment! But if you can't pull your legs up to the ledge, you won't be able to hold on forever!

Is this weird to think of survival? Perhaps, but at the end of the day, if the shit hits the fan, I want to know that I have basic movement skills to put me in a better position to survive!

The deskbound body

'Desk shoulders'

Most office-type work encourages a posture known as **upper crossed syndrome**. This involves:

- **Tight muscles:** Chest (pectorals) and upper neck/traps become tight from hunching forward.
- **Weak muscles:** Upper back muscles (rhomboids, lower traps) and deep neck flexors become lengthened and weak.

This imbalance causes the shoulder joint to move out of its optimal position, leading to impingement, instability, and overuse injuries. This program directly counteracts that imbalance and works to integrate preventative exercise for the other significant 'problem areas' that many of us develop over time, such as *anterior pelvic tilt* (see below).

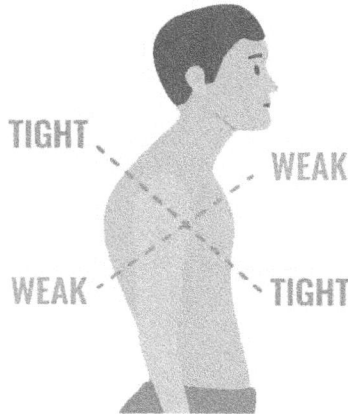

TIGHT

WEAK

WEAK

TIGHT

UPPER CROSSED SYNDROME

Quick tips when you're at your desk

1. **Ergonomics:** Ensure your monitor is at eye level and your keyboard allows your elbows to be at a 90-degree angle.

2. **Micro-breaks:** Every 30 minutes, stand up, roll your shoulders back, and stretch your neck. **The best posture is your next posture.**

3. **Scapular retractions:** Several times a day, sit tall and gently squeeze your shoulder blades together for 5 seconds. This "wakes up" the postural muscles.

'Desk hips' & the posterior chain

Prolonged sitting and lack of daily movement can also create a pattern of dysfunction in the lower body:

- **Tight & weak hip flexors:** As mentioned at the beginning of this chapter, your hips are constantly in a flexed (shortened) position, making the muscles tight. Because they are never fully lengthened or strengthened, they also become weak.

- **Gluteal amnesia:** Your glutes are inactive and lengthened while sitting. The brain essentially "forgets" how to fire them properly, leading to weakness.

- **Anterior dominance:** To compensate for weak glutes, the body relies on the muscles on the front of the legs (quadriceps) for movements like squatting and climbing stairs.

- **Tight hamstrings:** Weak glutes often cause the hamstrings to overwork and become chronically tight.

Quick tips when you're at your desk

1. **Walk around:** The most straightforward solution. Take calls while walking or get up every hour to walk to the water cooler.

2. **Desk glute squeezes:** While sitting, consciously squeeze your glutes hard for 5-10 seconds. Release and repeat. This helps re-establish the mind-muscle connection.

3. **Stand up, sit down:** Practice standing up from your chair and sitting back down slowly *without* using your hands. This is a functional bodyweight squat.

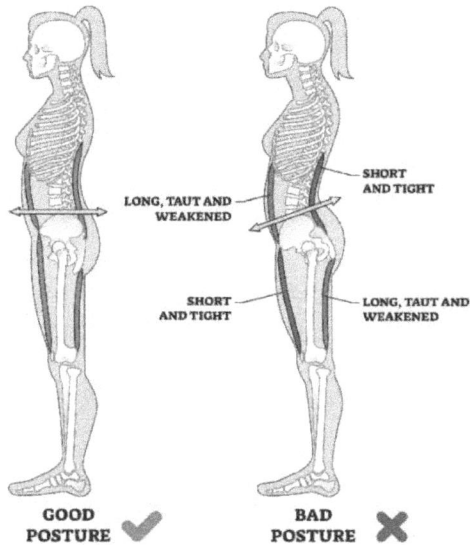

LONG, TAUT AND WEAKENED

SHORT AND TIGHT

SHORT AND TIGHT

LONG, TAUT AND WEAKENED

GOOD POSTURE

BAD POSTURE

The Core is a canister, not a crunch machine!

Think of your core as a 360-degree canister. The front (abs), sides (obliques), back (lower back muscles), top (diaphragm), and bottom (pelvic floor), along with deep abdominal muscles like the transversus abdominus, ubiquitous stabilisers and fixators like the quadratus lumborum, and even the hip flexors and glutes, all work together to create stability.

Traditional exercises like crunches only train one small part of this system (spinal flexion) and can sometimes worsen the slouched posture we're trying to fix. This program focuses on the core's primary job: resisting unwanted movement and creating a rigid, stable torso.

1. **"Draw in" your navel:** Throughout the day, practice gently pulling your belly button in towards your spine without holding your breath. This activates your deep transverse abdominis muscle, which acts like a natural corset for your spine.

2. **Belly breathing (diaphragmatic breathing):** Place a hand on your stomach. As you inhale through your nose, focus on making your hand rise before your chest does. This type of breathing properly engages your diaphragm, the "lid" of your core canister.

3. **Brace for action:** Before you pick up a box of printer paper or lift your luggage, consciously brace your core just like you would for a *Pallof Press*. Make this stability a real-world habit.

Yoga – an ancient way to put it all together

As part of my general routine, I typically do a short (less than 20 minutes) yoga session at the end of my working day (around 3:30 – 4:00 pm). This provides an active mobility session, incorporating breathing and mindfulness exercises, along with moves, stretches, and body activations to help alleviate the effects of hours spent sitting at a desk in front of a computer.

07

INJURIES & CHRONIC PAIN

As people who have seen more than a few decades of exercise, activity, and the rigours of life, the over-40 athlete has typically seen their fair share of injuries. Many of us also work around some degree of chronic pain in our lives.

An injury is explicitly related to an event. If you get injured, it's imperative to have the injury accurately diagnosed, treated, and perform the appropriate rehabilitation exercises to heal, remodel, and regain both mobility and strength in the affected area. This is obvious... so, if you're injured, see your doctor and a good physiotherapist. However, there are some other things you can do if you're injured to speed up the healing process (and to help prevent injuries in the future.

Injury is thought of as a purely mechanical phenomenon. In other words, you get hit by something (or you hit something!) and the physical trauma creates an injury, and there's little you can do about it. So, while the role of nutrition (and lifestyle) in rehabilitation from injury is intuitive, its role in preventing injuries and mitigating the severity of injury effects is drastically underappreciated.

The role of nutrition in rehabilitation is widely accepted, and improved nutrition is known to lead to faster recovery times.[15] However, its effects are underestimated during the acute injury phase and in the prevention of injury.[16]

What are some of the predictors of injury?

Many lifestyle-related factors are causally associated with the incidence of injury and its severity. These can include[17]:

- Body composition (relative muscle vs fat)
- Energy deficit
- Glycogen depletion
- Protein insufficiency
- Nutrient density (quality of nutrition)
- Vitamin D levels
- Lipid profile
- Hydration status

- Alcohol intake

Other likely predictors include:

- Immobility and improper warm-up and mobility work
- Stress
- Lack of sleep

Nutrition status and injury

Insufficient energy intake can lead to increased fatigue and favour catabolic over anabolic processes in the body (for example, the free testosterone to cortisol ratio). This might predispose someone to a greater risk of injury during sports and activities.

Once someone is injured, there is also a greater requirement (above baseline) for energy to fuel the recovery process. Energy requirements can increase by up to 20% after an injury, and this can rise to 50% greater following an injury or major surgery. It is important to note, however, that this is in addition to what would typically be required at rest.

Thus, the overall energy requirement may still be less than what was consumed during higher activity levels before the injury. Therefore, athletes should consume more energy than they would if they were sedentary (but often less than they did during competition).

Specific nutrients post-injury

A nutrient-rich diet, sufficient in fibre, vitamins, minerals, and secondary nutrients, is likely to aid recovery.[18]

Athletes should also make sure to consume at least 1.5 g of protein per kg of body weight per day to provide the amino acids necessary to rebuild damaged tissue. A lack of sufficient omega-3 fats can also reduce recovery *and* predispose someone to injury.[18]

Nutrition and brain injuries

Concussion and brain injury are common in many sports, including contact sports (rugby, fighting, and ice hockey), along with football (from repeated 'heading' of the ball) and resulting from bike or kayak crashes in endurance activities.

It is now known that the effects of brain injury can be mitigated through proper nutrition management,[19] and that this is not limited to the post-injury window, but that there may also be prophylactic effects of nutrition on concussion and brain injury.

Post-injury, fuelling damaged neurons is critical. Neurons may have a lessened ability to uptake glucose (their preferred fuel). They may also be at risk of hypoxic damage due to direct trauma and to the distortion of the blood-brain barrier, which can allow long-chain fatty acids to enter the brain. The importance of adequate fuel has been demonstrated in research on severe brain injuries in which every 10 calorie per kg decrease in intake was associated with a 30–40% increase in mortality rates.[20]

Ketogenic diets, ketones, and brain injuries

Due to distortions in the ability of neurons to adequately utilise glucose and the risk of hypoxic damage from the ingress of long-chain fatty acids, there is a potential role for ketones and ketogenic diets in mitigating the effects of brain injuries, which warrants further research.[21] In fact, astrocytes of the brain are known to 'scavenge' fatty acids to convert to ketones to both reduce the risk of hypoxic damage and to provide fuel for neurons.[22]

Ketones are protective against the effects of ischemia (loss of blood supply to tissue),[23,24] and cell damage caused by hypoglycaemia.[25] Ketones are also known to modulate the glutamate-GABA ratio in the brain and nervous system,[26] and inflammation,[27] thereby reducing excitotoxicity (protecting neurons from this cytotoxic damage) and improving the structure and function of glial cells.[28]

It is essential to avoid the temptation to increase glucose availability (through high-carbohydrate diets) post-injury, as excitotoxicity is exacerbated by excessive carbohydrate intake and rebound hypoglycaemia but is mitigated by ketones and a ketogenic diet.[29] Interestingly, ketones also reduce oxidative stress in the brain and increase brain-derived neurotrophic factor (BDNF), which helps the brain to repair itself.[30]

Lion's Mane for the brain?

Various fungi, in particular Lion's Mane mushroom (*Hericium erinaceus*), show promise as treatments for brain injury due to their neurogenic properties. Lion's Mane has been shown to increase 'Nerve Growth Factor' (NGF),[31] which helps nerves and brain cells to grow and repair,[32-37] an effect not observed in other medicinal fungi, such as Eringi, Maitake, and Himematsutake.[38]

Commonly used supplements for injury prevention and management

Fish oil

While fish oil has not been demonstrated to improve sports performance, omega-3 fatty acids are essential for proper immune and inflammatory modulation in athletes.[39] Acute exercise increases reactive oxygen species (ROS) and inflammatory markers, and reduces phagocytic activity of white blood cells. DHA-rich fish oil has been shown to reduce ROS and inflammation, and improve neutrophil integrity and activity.[40] In animal research, it has been demonstrated that fish oil can restore dopamine release post-brain injury.[41]

Fish oil also significantly modulates inflammation post-brain injury in humans,[42] and results in significantly reduced time in intensive care, and total hospital admission time.[43]

Collagen

Collagen hydrolysate has a range of anti-inflammatory and joint-supporting properties.[44,45] When taken orally, collagen hydrolysate peptides can enter the bloodstream,[46,47] and accumulate in cartilage, where they increase the synthesis of connective tissue.[48] As little as 1200 mg per day of collagen has been shown to significantly improve joint pain after six months.[49] While a 10 g dose of collagen taken daily reduces pain and improves joint mobility and function in people with arthritis,[50,51] and reduces joint pain and inflammation in athletes.[52]

Glucosamine

Some beneficial effects of glucosamine supplementation have been observed in osteoarthritis, and recent research suggests that glucosamine may help reduce collagen degradation in endurance athletes.[53-55] However, several studies have shown that glucosamine supplementation (~1500 mg per day) *did not* significantly reduce knee pain after 28 days.[56,57] However, there was a significant improvement in joint range of motion compared to the control.[57]

Take-home messages

To reduce the risk of injury

- Ensure appropriate energy intake
- Ensure optimal protein intake (goal dependent)
- Ensure adequate micronutrient intake – consider a multinutrient supplement
- Ensure adequate sun exposure (without burning! Consider vitamin D intake as part of supplement regimen)
- Encourage optimal, healthy body composition and metabolic status
- Ensure the athlete is adequately hydrated – 2 glasses on rising, 2 litres through the day, 1 litre per hour of exercise
- Reduce alcohol intake to healthy norms (i.e., <3-5 standard drinks per week)
- Encourage mindfulness practice
- Put in place sleep hygiene practices to encourage optimal sleep duration (i.e., 7-9.5 hours per night) and quality

If you're injured

- Adjust energy to meet activity
- Consume a 'carb-appropriate' diet
- Ensure optimal protein intake (goal dependent)
- Ensure adequate micronutrient intake – consider a multinutrient supplement
- Ensure adequate sun exposure (without burning!) Consider vitamin D intake as part of a supplement regimen
- Encourage optimal, healthy body composition and metabolic status

- Ensure the athlete is adequately hydrated – 2 glasses on rising, 2 litres through the day, 1 litre per hour of exercise
- Reduce alcohol intake to healthy norms (i.e., <3-5 standard drinks per week)
- Encourage mindfulness practice
- Put in place sleep hygiene practices to encourage optimal sleep duration (i.e., 7-9.5 hours per night) and quality
- Consider supplementation: multi, fish oil, collagen, glucosamine/chondroitin, for brain: Lion's Mane, ketones, MCTs

Chronic pain

Chronic pain is a different beast altogether. While past injuries *can* result in immobility, changes in range of motion, and may cause pain during movements or through specific ranges of motion, nagging chronic pain shows little association with particular pathologies. In other words, past injuries or even present physical maladies (if not serious) usually have little to do with chronic, ongoing, and frequently presenting pain, and these have more to do with lifestyle, diet, emotions, thought patterns, and other lifestyle and psychosocial factors.

Of course, you should always rule out any more serious reasons for pain, and it's vital if you have ongoing pain to have it thoroughly investigated by your physician and attend any referrals they recommend. Still, you might find that your pain is not pathological...

Chronic pain is considered a condition in and of itself because it lasts longer than the injury and healing time from which it resulted, or is found without an explaining pathology.[58] Around 20% of people worldwide experience chronic pain.[58]

The most common chronic pain is low-back pain, and the evidence suggests that there is no association between chronic back pain and spinal pathologies. In other words, there are around the same number of people with pathology and pain as there are without pathology and pain and with pathology but without pain! This shows clearly that the 'usual suspects' of herniated disks, disk bulges, joint narrowing of the vertebrae and other purported 'causes' of back pain are not so. In fact, the strongest association with low-back pain is fear. This and other psycho-social factors are now considered to be the primary reasons for the ongoing expression of low-back pain.

Dr John Sarno coined a term to describe the condition of this non-physical pain syndrome: *tension myositis* or *tension myoneural syndrome* (TMS), in which the culprit behind back and other chronic muscular and joint pain is 'tension' provided primarily by psycho-emotional factors and, in part, fear of the pain and the supposedly related pathologies themselves.[59]

While this syndrome is not accepted in the medical community and there are several mechanistic issues with Sarno's theory, it has become universally accepted that pathology has little if any association with most chronic pain and that pain results from a confluence of factors, including, but not limited to:

- Emotional trauma
- Other mental and emotional states of tension
- Nutrition
- Past injuries, posture, and other physical factors, although these may play a lesser role than the psychosocial and psycho-emotional causes of pain.

How to deal with chronic pain

Firstly, it's crucial to rule out any physical cause of pain. Serious illnesses, including autoimmune conditions, cancer, and cardiometabolic conditions, can result in pain, and there may also be underlying injuries or physiological problems that are either causing or contributing to your pain. If these are ruled out, though, it is important to remember that your pain is not likely to be caused by pathology.

To free oneself from pain, introspective exercises can be highly beneficial. If you experience chronic pain, or if you have a relapse of pain or more serious pain:

- Remind yourself that *my pain is not necessarily pathological*
- Ask yourself, "Why am I experiencing this pain?"
  - o Consider what 'else' is going on in your life: Have you slept poorly the night or nights before? Have you experienced a stressful event?

Are you overtrained?

Has something triggered past trauma to arise?

- Ask yourself, "Why am I experiencing pain overall?"
  - o Do you have unresolved trauma?
  - o Are you in a relationship, environment, or lifestyle that is counter to your ethos, your perceived 'life purpose', or that is in some way physically or mentally damaging?

You may find that the mere awareness that your pain is not necessarily resulting from pathology (you're not broken!) can have an enormous effect on the severity of the chronic pain, and recognising other psychosocial factors that play into your pain can help you to resolve those underlying issues and free yourself.

Of course, if you need help with past trauma or current life situations that are affecting your health and well-being, seek out a qualified and credible mental health professional to guide you.

A case for slow

Having experienced numerous injuries, I've realised the value of slow and controlled movements. This might be a 'duh' moment for many of you reading this, but hear me out…

Often, as people obsessed with strength and performance, we focus on power and explosiveness. On balance, I think developing and retaining the ability to move (and move load) quickly as we age is a critical part of remaining healthy and functional, but there are times (and post-injury is one) that we want to really slow down movements, focusing on practising perfect positioning.

An interesting aspect of this is that it typically allows for micro-adjustments during a lift, helping maintain appropriate positioning and enabling a larger pain-free range of motion. So, while explosive training is critical to overall health and performance, so is slow and controlled training.

Example: Try taking a full 5 seconds to raise and lower the weight (or your body) under complete control.

A case for bodyweight

In addition to slow training, bodyweight training is an excellent adjunct to post-injury rehabilitation, returning from chronic fatigue or illness, or at any time!

While many people dismiss bodyweight training as limited because, at some point, one will be doing too many repetitions to improve strength or hypertrophy optimally, it's clear that these individuals haven't explored the various advanced progressions of bodyweight exercises, such as handstand pushups, single-leg squats, advanced bridges, single-arm pullups, and more.

08

TRAINING BY CLIFF

I employ a variety of styles in my training, and my workouts and programs vary based on my sleep levels, stress levels, other commitments, and what I'm currently reading. I tend to gravitate between low-volume, high-frequency training with short durations and longer, less frequent sessions. Overall, looking back over the years, I have trained with weights (30 and counting), achieving my best results from relatively short, intense, and frequent workouts. And now that I'm older, I tend to find that slightly longer intervals between body parts or movements (as discussed in the previous chapter) work best for me.

Terminology

Various abbreviations are used in training circles. While these vary by coach, we have used the following standard abbreviations in the programs in this and later chapters, which are commonly used in the industry:

Term	Abbreviation
Barbell	BB
Dumbbell	DB
Kettlebell	KB
Single-leg	SL
Single-arm	SA

Full body training

One day per week

One day is, by nature, the least you can strength train in any given week. Most authorities would suggest that it's not enough to optimise your strength and for health, the evidence suggests that you should perform at least two strength training sessions per week.[60] However, whether one day per week *can* be effective is far more nuanced.

While a greater frequency (even when volume is equated) is likely to be marginally more effective for strength and hypertrophy than a lesser frequency, total volume and progressive overload are the primary factors for improving strength and gaining and retaining muscle.

If nothing else, something is better than nothing, and if one can commit fully to one effective strength training session per week, it is far better than failing to complete a plan with more training days. Everyone's lives, schedules, and recovery ability are different, and a one-day-per-week program might work wonders for you. However, if you have time to train more, then do it.

Since volume and overload are key to progress, you should perform a one-day-per-week program on the day when you have the most time and flexibility. For most people, this typically occurs on the weekend (or another day off if you're on a non-traditional work schedule). That way, your training can be longer, allowing adequate work volume and rest periods.

Extreme minimalist

Exercise	Options	Work sets	Repetitions	Rest
BB Military Press	DB, KB, or Handstand Pushups	4	6-15	1-3 min
Pullups	Table Rows, Chest-supported Rows	4	6-15	
BB Back Squats	Front Squats (BB, KB, DB), Deadlifts, Pistol Squats, or another bodyweight squat	4	6-15	

In this plan, the trainer receives a 'minimum effective dose' of compound movements, as suggested in the recent review by

Iverson and colleagues,[10] in one relatively short workout per week. The set and rep schemes enable a crossover of strength and hypertrophy, provided there is sufficient overall loading and volume for both outcomes. If you are extremely time-constrained, consider reducing the rest periods to one minute and feel free to superset the presses and pulls.

On the other hand, if you have more time on your given training day, extend the rest period to 3 minutes, which should allow greater loading due to reduced cumulative fatigue. As always, train to a comfortable repetition maximum, keeping a rep or two 'in the bank,' and focus on increasing the load you use over the course of a training cycle.

The 3-5 Program

The 3-5 program is one of my favourites. Many people have claimed to invent the 3-5 workout, but it has been used in some form and under different names since the explosion of strength and physical culture in the 1930s to 1950s. More recently, fantastic iterations of *3-5* have been published by strength gurus like Pavel and Dan John.

A plan I have used (and recommended) frequently since the late 1990s is simple in the extreme.

Perform 3-5 exercises for 3-5 sets of 3-5 reps, 3-5 times per week, resting 3-5 minutes between sets...

Simple huh?

Which exercises should you use?

You can choose any exercises for this, but it makes sense to focus on the key movement patterns: squat (and/or hip hinge), press, row, and hip hinge and add 1-2 assistance exercises. For example, a snatch or clean variation, a back squat, a press variation, kettlebell swings, and either a triceps or bicep exercise would fit the bill for most people.

Depending on your focus, here are a few other examples.

Powerlifting

- Squat
- Bench Press
- Deadlift
- Chest-supported Rows or heavy Cheat Curls
- Triceps Extensions

Olympic weightlifting

- Barbell Snatch
- Barbell Clean and Jerk (perform these as 'strength practice, focused 100% on form)
- Back Squat
- Overhead Press
- Power Clean

All-Round Weightlifting

- Overhead Press
- Single-arm Barbell Snatch

- Power Clean / Power Jerk
- Back Squat
- Floor Press

Strongman

- Front Squat
- Single-arm Shoulder Press
- Deadlift
- Ball or Stone Lifts
- Loaded Carries (Farmer's Walks)

The variety of plans is endless. Ensure that you cover all the major movement patterns throughout your training year. If you have weak points (such as retraction/rowing/shoulder position), ensure you work on exercises that target those areas.

Whole body, two-way split performed 2-6 times per week

When most people think of split programs, they think of splitting up body parts, but another way to split is to use different movement patterns or exercises on alternate training days. This enables frequent training of body parts, which is likely to be most effective for both strength and hypertrophy while also providing novelty and relative reductions in loading. This is also a fantastic way to train if you need to incorporate several specific lifts into your plan (for example, if you are a competitive All-Round Weightlifter).

Some of my favourite varieties of this style of plan are:

Day 1.

Exercise	Work sets	Repetitions	Rest
BB Power Snatch	8	1	1-3 min
BB Back Squat	5	5	
BB Bench Press	4	4-8	

Day 2.

Exercise	Work sets	Repetitions	Rest
BB Clean & Push Press	3	3+3	1-3 min
BB Front Squat	4	8	
DB Military Press	4	8	

Push-Pull Split performed 2-6 times per week

Day 1.

Exercise	Work sets	Repetitions	Rest
DB Military Press	3	8	1-3 min
BB Cheat Curl	3	6	
KB Floor Press	4	4-8	
Alternating DB Curl	2	10-20	
KB Overhead Tricep Extension	2	10-20	

Day 2.

Exercise	Work sets	Repetitions	Rest
BB Back Squat	5	5	1-3 min
Chest-supported DB Rows	4	8	
KB Swings (Russian 'Hard Style')	4	10	
Pullups	4	Tmax	

Upper-Lower split performed 2-6 times per week

Day 1.

Exercise	Work sets	Repetitions	Rest
BB Military Press	5	5	1-3 min
Power Clean from the knee to Push Press	3	3+3	
DB Bench Press	3	8	
BB Curls	4	6	

Day 2.

Exercise	Work sets	Repetitions	Rest
BB Power Snatch	5	2	1-3 min
BB Back Squat	5	5	
Abs (whatever you desire!)	4	10	

One lift per day

For most of my training life, I have focused on whole-body (or 2-way splits), as my primary goal has always been strength development for competition or as an adjunct to martial arts. Apart from periods in my teens and early twenties, I have typically eschewed bodybuilding-type splits or programs that focus on a body part or movement trained infrequently (i.e., once per week). However, that changed when we had a baby...

Initially, my training when we first had our little guy was *awesome!* He slept like a dream, and during my early morning training sessions, I made them as hard and long as I desired while he and my partner slept. That all changed when he had his first sleep regression, and after waking (around 5 or 6 times some nights), the last thing I wanted to do was an extended full-body program with several of the 'big guys' (like cleans, squats, and presses) all included in the one session.

I experimented with a return to more bodybuilding-style training, exploring programs such as Jim Wendler's 5-3-1 and Dan John's One Exercise Per Day plans. The flexibility in these types of plans was just what the doctor ordered for an underslept Dad.

Example

	M	T	W	Th	F	Sa
Focus activity	BJJ	Overhead press	BJJ	Squat	Bench	Deadlift
Assistance work	Yoga	Bench assistance	Yoga	Squat/ Row assistance*	Overhead Press assistance	Deadlift/ Row assistance

*I usually just squat on my squat day. Sometimes, I'll add pullups, rows, and some additional squat or lunge variations.

**I mostly tend to press off the floor for two reasons: 1) Shoulder injuries... and 2) It has a good transfer to both grappling and All-Round weightlifting (in which the pullover and push or pullover and press are often performed as competition lifts).

Cross-training

To my mind, for the over-40 athlete, the best cross-training is doing something you love. I tend to go through phases of running, HIIT (as part of or instead of assistance work), and more metabolic-conditioning-style strongman work, depending on my mood. However, one consistent aspect of my cross-training and conditioning regimen is grappling. Grappling (catch-wrestling and Brazilian Jiu Jitsu) is one of the most challenging workouts I have ever done, and the fact that you are wrestling another human (who, incidentally, is trying to either tear a limb off you or choke you unconscious!) provides a level that you need to rise to.

If you know, you know...

Bodyweight training

Bodyweight training can be an equally effective mode for anyone looking to become or maintain a strong, mobile, healthy body. Sure, you're not going to win the Olympics in Weightlifting or place in Powerlifting competitions unless you're training with weights... but that's not because the various weight lifts make you strong per se (of course they do...) but that they allow you to be strong generally and specifically strong in the movement patterns of the lifts you train for. However, if you don't *need* to be strong in a snatch, jerk, squat, deadlift, or bench press, then bodyweight training can provide all the stimulus you need.

One advantage of bodyweight training is that progressions are, by nature, very limiting. So, it is more difficult to rush into loads that put you at risk, and, for whatever reason, (and this might just be my experience) bodyweight training is also very good for improving total body tension and control and is, at least for people getting back into training, often superior for these outcomes to barbell training. However, it doesn't need to be all one way or another; combining bodyweight and external load training is a definite win-win.

Example bodyweight progressions

Exercise	Progression 1	2	3	4	5
Pulls	Table rows	Self-assisted Pullups	Negative Pullups	Pullups	SA Pullups
Squats	Bodyweight ½ Squat	BW full Squat	Narrow Squat	One-legged Squat	'Pistol' squats
Pushes	Pushups against the wall	Pushups from knees	Pushups	Close-grip Pushups	SA Pushups
Bridges	Short Bridges	Single-leg Bridges	Straight Bridges	Full Bridge	Wrestler's Bridge
Abs	Plank on knees	Plank	Side Plank	Plank to Side Plank (Plank Rotation)	Ab Rollouts

Perform as many repetitions as you are *easily able to*. When you can do 20-30 repetitions of an exercise easily and with total control, move on to the next progression.

Example hybrid training

As my son got a little older, he wasn't so amenable to sitting in his playpen while I lifted in the morning (both my kids now train with me in the morning).

So, I adapted my training to the following:

AM – Mobility and Bodyweight

One set (to an easy daily 'max') of:

- Pike Arches
- Postural lunges
- Pushups
- Surf slides
- Standing bodyweight rows
- Squat progressions

Lunch time

3-5 sets of 3-5:

- Barbell squats
- Kettlebell military press
- Floor KB press
- KB one-arm rows
- Rotational ab work

Cardio-crossover training

Cardio-crossover is the term I use for everything from 'true' cardio like Zone 2 through to HIIT and AGT, which have been mentioned earlier in the book.

I typically use cardio as a 'finisher' at the end of a workout, before lunch or at the end of my working day, or as 'active recovery' on off days. I light how I feel guides the intensity of my cardio, and since I already engage in a lot of high-intensity work in BJJ, I usually gravitate towards short bouts of Zone 2 and AGT.

Sample Zone 2 circuit

Unless I am going out for a very brisk walk, or even more rarely a jog, my 'go to' Zone 2 activity is doing circuits of light kettlebell and/or mace and Indian club training. Here is a sample session (for 15-30 min)

- Light Indian club swinging – inside-out circles, simultaneous and alternating
- Lunges with clubs
- Indian club Russian-style swings
- Clubbell crucifix squats
- 1 arm mace swinging – full circles, each side
- Mace lunges with a twist

The absolute key with the circuit above is that you are constantly moving to preserve an elevated heart rate, but also that you can sustain a conversation (the 'Talk Test') during the entire duration to remain in Zone 2.

Feel free to experiment with any exercises for these types of circuits, but remember to keep them light, flowing, and within the bounds of the Talk Test.

Sample AGT workout

One of my go-to AGT workouts is loosely based on the AXE training protocol by Pavel Tsatsouline. It involves repeating just two exercises, pushups and kettlebell swings, alternated for 10 explosive, submaximal reps, 'on the minute'.

This provides around 50 seconds of rest for each work period, emphasising explosiveness and using loads that preserve maximal speed. Consequently, there is no risk of nearing muscular failure. For anything from five to 30 minutes, alternate the following every minute, on the minute:

- Pushups x 10 explosive reps
- Rest until the next minute
- Kettlebell swings x 10 (Russian style, explosive – lockout hard at the top with a 'double brace' of the abs and glutes)
- Rest until the next minute and repeat

And more!

I haven't covered various bodybuilding style splits here, which can also have enormous value for the over-40 athlete.

If you are interested in accessing more training programs by me, along with customised coaching options, check out: **www.cliffharvey.com/coaching**

09

TRAINING BY DAZ

I somewhat squandered my peak training years, taking a 20-year-old body that was already a little beat up from martial arts and poorly guided gym training, overseas for a decade of partying, low-paying jobs, and 3rd-world travel.

By my 30s, I was back on track, though, and I consider this decade to be my best in terms of sheer strength, capacity, and competitive drive. That last point is important because now that my goals have shifted away from competition and the pursuit of numbers on a scoreboard, my perception of what it means to be fit has also shifted. Now, a newly minted 50-year-old (at the time of writing), I'm not as capable of the physical feats I once was, but thanks to a decade of much more intentional (vs intense) training, I also have longer and better sleep, get twice as many outdoor steps per day, and have more muscle mass.

The low back and shoulder pain that plagued me on and off for almost 30 years has gone. The other significant difference is that

I still train regularly (I do something physical most days), albeit with reduced volume.

This had numerous positive effects:

- Decreased stress/cortisol and improved recovery capacity (critical as we lose this ability with age).
- No limping around the next day with brutal muscle soreness (you never want to have to tell your kid you were too tender to play with them after leg day...).
- Decreased risk of injury (jacking up your back on a deadlift 1RM might be a twisted badge of honour in your 20s, but it's a liability and feels embarrassing in your 40s).

I improved my motivation and consistency. Training every day meant it was just what I did, and it became much easier to fit into my schedule. Also, because I wasn't killing myself in the gym, it wasn't hard to get it done, no matter what, even if I had had a poor sleep or a tough day in the office.

One of my clients, for whom the lightbulb finally went off after numerous conversations about longevity vs performance, messaged me with the excited zeal of the newly converted, "I've realised that I just need to train more, but do less!" he said.

Specifically, he meant that he had realised that three or four long gruelling workouts per week, alternated with the inevitable days of sore muscles, aching joints and low energy, was not practical (or fun) when juggling a stressful job, kids, poor sleep, and commuting, not to mention being a decade older. Instead, he tried exercising every day, but in a sensible amount and with a sensible effort. Suddenly, he felt better; aches and pains cleared up, his energy improved throughout the day, his mood improved, his motivation increased, and his sleep quality improved.

We're built to move daily, but if you have a desk job and drive to work, you might be getting fewer than 1,000 steps on a rest day. And it doesn't matter what you did before that rest day, 'sitting is the new smoking' as some experts like to say controversially. An hour of movement per day is still only 4% of the week, so you mustn't let a day go by without doing something.

We mentioned minimum effective dose earlier in the book. The minimum amount of work needed to create some adaptation above baseline. We also have a *maximum effective dose*, but training close to this threshold is only possible with the corresponding maximum recovery capacity, which is rare to find among anyone who isn't a professional athlete.

Unless you're willing to quit your job and move back in with your parents, you can't expect to benefit from training for training's sake. Instead, you're a professional human being, and if you want to be the best in the world at managing work, family, friends, hobbies and health, the minimum effective training dose is where your focus should lie.

Also, if you're anything like me, your attention is often pulled in multiple directions by the above elements. It's all too easy to find yourself running out of time to complete the entire workout you'd planned, or worse, working out while also sending emails between sets and texting your partner about who is doing the kids' sports pickup. This is where short, sharp workouts, which use the clock to keep us on point are incredibly helpful.

Here are a few examples of 'bang for your buck' workout programs that have you in and out of the gym in 30-45 minutes, and sometimes even less.

OTM workouts

OTM is short for 'on the minute.' Set a clock to beep every 60 seconds and use it to stay focused, efficient, and effective. The rest periods are short in this program, and as such, you're moving fairly constantly, meaning you get a lot done in a short period of time. This also means you must work with light to moderate loads, which requires a less extensive warm-up and a lower risk of injury. Finally, you'll get a fantastic muscle-building pump as well as a conditioning effect.

The example shows four exercises, each as two supersets. Perform a set of A1 at the start of minute 1, then a set of A2 at the beginning of minute 2, then back to A1, for 3 to 6 total sets of each (depending on time available and your instincts for your max effective dose). Take a 2-4 minute rest and then repeat for B1 and B2.

Progression

Progressive overload means increasing the demands on the muscles, joints, and the cardiovascular system over time as you get used to the initial stimulus, such that you are constantly improving.

Adding more weight to the bar is the default progression in the weight room for most, but, as our example of Milo illustrates, this can't be sustained forever. So, in addition to considering adding an extra kilo to the bar next week, you could do one more rep.

This can often be an easier route than adding more load, especially if you're training at home with minimal equipment. E.g., eight squats on week 1, nine on week 2, 10 on week 3, then 11, then 12. THEN you go back to eight reps, but add some extra load and begin the process again.

Other methods you can use besides reps and weight are:

- increased range of motion (can you squat deeper, or pull up higher each week?)
- tempo (slowing down the rep, particularly on the lowering phase to increase tension on the muscle)

- adding more volume (e.g. three supersets on week one, four supersets on week two, etc.)
- increasing mind-muscle connection (may sound a bit woo, but trying to feel the muscle working and your intent to make the contraction stronger really works!)

DAY 1	Exercise	Reps	Notes
A1	Squats	8-12	load anyhow: goblet, front, back, double DB/KB
A2	Pull-ups	4-8	
B1	Side Plank Hip Lifts	8-10	
B2	Bicep Curls	10-15	

DAY 2	Reps	Exercise
A1	8-12	Romanian Deadlifts
A2	10-15	Pushups
B1	10-12	V-ups
B2	10-15	DB Overhead Tricep Extensions

DAY 3	Reps	Exercise	Equipment/Load
A1	12-16	Reverse Lunges	goblet, front, back, double DB/KB
A2	8-10	Bent-over Rows	BB, double or single KB/DB
B1	12-15	DB Lateral Raises	
B2	10-15	Bicep Curls	

DAY 4	Reps	Exercise
A1	8-12	Sumo Deadlifts
A2	8-12	Strict Press
B1	8-12	Hanging Knee Raises
B2	8-12	Skull Crushers

AMRAP ladders

I love these kinds of workouts because the warm-up is built right in via the lower-rep sets. By the time it gets tough, your heart rate is up, and you've got a sweat on. Conversely, only the last few minutes of the workout are truly challenging. This is a good thing before or after a long day in the office, a physical job, or wrangling kids.

You have enough stress as it is, and thus these ladders tick the box of a minimum effective dose - just enough to make you feel good and be better tomorrow, rather than being beaten down, sore, and unable to sleep because you're still in fight-or-flight mode from some crazy high-intensity intervals.

Example upper body workout

- 2-4-6-8-10-12...etc as far as possible in 10 min
- KB or DB Gorilla Rows
- Push Ups

Example lower body workout

- For 10 min
- 2-4-6...etc.
- Russian Swings
- 1-2-3...etc.
- Goblet Squats

Example full body workout

- 2-4-6... etc for 10 min
- Dumbbell Burpee
- DB Reverse Lunge
- DB Hang power clean and push press

You can progress these workouts by simply trying to get further up the ladder next time. At some point, you could increase the weight you're using, or you can make it a 12-minute ladder instead of 10, then 14, etc.

A longer 20-minute session works well with a cardio option added to your strength moves, e.g.:

- 2-4-6-8-10-12...etc as far as possible in 20 mins
- KB or DB Gorilla Rows
- Pushups
- 5-10 calorie Row after each round

Density training

These circuits are a favourite of mine; they offer a great way to use the timer to keep yourself focused, retain a strength and hypertrophy emphasis, while maintaining the overall intensity to a manageable level. Also, great if you find yourself twiddling your thumbs (or worse, scrolling your thumbs) during long rest periods.

Here's a two-part full-body workout. You're working for 16 minutes, but the focus is on load and movement quality, not racing the clock. Take short breaks as needed.

A: For 16 mins

- 8 Sumo Deadlifts, increase weight each round
- 8/side Kettlebell Strict Press
- 8 Goblet Cossack squats, alternating

B: For 10 mins

- 15 Ring Rows

- 15 Pushups
- 30m/side Suitcase Carry

50s &100s

This high-rep, 'get it done & get on with the day' approach is always my fallback when life is really trying to trip me up. There are two ways to tackle this:

Morning hundy

As soon as you get out of bed, accumulate 50 - 100 reps of 1-to-2 movements.

E.g., 5-10 squats + 5-10 pushups x 10 rounds

Or slot in some prehab work for those tight hips and shoulders.

E.g., 6-10 lateral Romanian lunges + 10-15 banded pull-aparts

If you feel up to a bit more intensity, then you could chunk it into bigger sets and challenge yourself a bit more. For example, try to complete 50 push-ups in just three sets with minimal rest between, or perhaps one single set of walking lunges or Russian swings for as many reps as possible.

Even if you plan to work out later in the day, this little session not only fires you up for the morning but also boosts your metabolic rate and motivates you to make better choices throughout the day.

If your later workout falls through, it's not a total failure because you've already done something!

OTH (on the hour)

This method I used to great effect when in the hospital while my wife gave birth. There were plenty of times when I was just in the way, so I'd head out into the corridor every hour and bang out a few reps of pushups, squats, lunges, handstand holds or hollow rocks. Flights of stairs were also a fantastic addition to this method, and by the end of the day, I'd easily managed 100 reps of 1-2 movements, if not closer to 300 on a couple of long days!

To keep me from getting behind on what is typically a crazy day, I will set 10 alarms on my phone, from say, 8 am until 5 pm, and when each goes off, I take a couple of minutes to myself and accumulate a few more reps.

For more programs and coaching by Daz, go to **https://www.darrenellis.coach/**

125

10

NUTRITION

The food we eat provides the building blocks for creating tissue and chemical messengers within the body, as well as the substrate used to replenish our cellular energy. Thus, it's a critical component of health. We all understand this (hence the multi-billion-dollar diet industry!), but implementing great nutrition is easier said than done.

Unlike exercise, which can drastically improve health with just a few hours of highly effective training per week, eating is something we do (and think about) several times a day, making it far more challenging to remain 'on track'.

Add to that the 'psychosocial milieu' within which food is tied up with society, culture, self-image, body dysmorphias, enjoyment, and emotions, and we have an extraordinarily complex area to work with!

Unfortunately, nutrition has also become over-complicated. Due to ongoing (and I believe unnecessary) 'diet wars' between low-carb and low-fat, vegan and carnivore, paleo, and food pyramid, etc., we tend to focus on which 'diet' works best rather than on the key components of healthy nutrition, irrespective of 'diet.'

*So, let's leave all the **shoulds** and **should nots** behind and focus instead on the key and fundamental concepts and strategies of healthy nutrition that 99.99% of nutrition authorities agree on (sorry, carnivores!)*

Concepts & strategies

Eat mostly natural, unrefined foods

Time and again, when we examine studies purporting to show the superiority of low-fat or low-carb, vegan or vegetarian, Paleo, or any other diet, we see that high-performing diets consistently focus on natural, unrefined foods and the consumption of fewer ultra-processed foods.

What about the 'naturalistic fallacy'

You'll notice above that I didn't shy away from using the term 'natural.' Some of you reading this might think that this is an example of the *naturalistic fallacy* or, more precisely, an *appeal to nature.* "The naturalistic fallacy is the idea that what is found in nature is good" (Steven Pinker), and conversely, that human-made or synthetic things are 'bad' or morally inferior. Natural does not necessarily mean good or better. There are plenty of natural things that will kill you very quickly (try chowing down on a Death Cap mushroom...).

Natural is also challenging to define, as commonly pointed out by scientists opposed to the use of the word in the field of nutrition sciences. For example, are the vegetables we commonly eat 'natural', given that they have been selectively bred for millennia and in their standard forms are found nowhere in nature? Is beef 'natural' given that there are no truly wild cattle?

These are all interesting debates; however, people understand what I mean when I say 'natural.' The word evokes thoughts, feelings, and imagery that people can relate to and understand. So, in the interests of getting results rather than pontificating from the sidelines, I'm happy to use terms that people understand.

Prioritise protein and vegetables

You're made from protein. Every cell, tissue, and organ in the body is built on a scaffold of proteins produced from the amino acids that we derive from protein in food. So, protein is critical as the foundation of your nutrition.

Vegetables provide additional vitamins, minerals, secondary nutrients that support the body's antioxidant status, cellular fuelling, and epigenetic signalling, and gut-supporting fibres and resistant starches.

While the carnivore crowd eschew them, almost all of us, virtually all the time, benefit from the addition of plentiful amounts and varieties of vegetables to our diet.

Eat carbohydrates according to your goals, activity levels, and metabolic state

The most significant debate in nutrition in recent times has been around the value and utility of carbohydrates in the diet, and because it is related to this debate, the quantity of fat we should consume.

To provide clarity to this debate, we can look at the roles of these nutrients in the body. As mentioned previously, protein provides the structure of the body (and little in the way of fuel provision), including being the building blocks for amino acid-derived hormones (like epinephrine, norepinephrine, and dopamine). Protein provides essential amino acids that the body cannot create.

Fat provides both structure (as a building block of steroid hormones, cell membranes, and other tissues) and fuel. Fat, in fact, is our primary fuel as it provides the bulk of our fuel provision at rest and during low-intensity activity. Fat also provides essential fatty acids (which the body cannot produce) and conditionally essential fats that help support hormone regulation and reduce the risk of overreaching and overtraining.

Carbohydrates, on the other hand, are not technically 'essential,' as glucose (the usable 'unit' of carbohydrate) can be produced in the body from amino acids (protein) and glycerol (from fats) and is mainly used for fuel and not within structures. However, it is the primary fuel for the brain and nervous system, as well as for higher-intensity exercise types. Therefore, we can consider it to be 'conditionally essential,' as we will benefit more or less, depending on our activity demands and our ability to use carbohydrate fuel effectively.

So, what do the roles of the macronutrients tell us?

1. **We should prioritise protein** as it provides the essential amino acids and conditionally essential amino acids necessary to build and maintain structures within the body.
2. **We should consume fat** in at least sufficient amounts to preserve hormonal integrity and more if we don't utilise carbohydrate as effectively or if we adhere better to a lower-carb way of eating.
3. **Carbohydrates should make up 'the rest'** of our energy allotment, as our activity volume and intensity will dictate this. Thus, we can consume enough carbohydrate to provide the glycogen (stored carbohydrate) to fuel our exercise bouts.

Choose meals over snacks

At the time of writing, with over 27 years of experience in fitness and health practice, I've noticed a common theme: overall, people tend to achieve far superior results when they focus on eating quality meals and eliminate snacks. Now, I'm not saying that no one should snack. If snacking works well for you, then fill your boots...

However, the reality is that for many people, snacking leads to a poorer quality diet, typically higher in refined foods and lower in protein, vegetables, and essential fats, compared to focusing on quality meals. Additionally, it causes many people to find themselves in the 'nowhere land' of dissatisfaction, which can lead to craving-driven eating – seldom a recipe for success!

Evidence suggests a strong link between snacking behaviours, poorer food choices and increased obesity rates.[61] I have seen stark evidence for this effect. For some clients, the one thing that worked in the long term wasn't calorie counting, step counting, 'if it fits your macros,' or any other diet – it was simply to stop snacking.

Eat when you're (*actually*) hungry, until you're (*actually*) full

This strategy complements the one above. There is no evidence that eating frequently and forcing yourself to eat throughout the day offers any benefits. Because snacking and 'grazing' behaviours are detrimental for many people, it's better to eat when you're hungry and stop when you're full.

If you are eating a diet based primarily on natural, unrefined foods, you'll naturally slip into a pattern of eating that may range from 1 to 6 meals per day, tailored to your individual needs.

For most people, the 'sweet spot' is 2-4 meals per day.

This rule also applies to specific meals. For example, if you're not hungry first thing in the morning...then don't eat breakfast! Eat when you first feel hungry...and make sure that each meal is a good, balanced one. Just bear in mind that the fewer meals you eat, the more protein you will need to include at each meal to optimise your protein intake, and you might be at greater risk of micronutrient insufficiencies. You should never sacrifice protein intake to reduce meal frequency.

The question arises, "How much should I eat?" and without overcomplicating the issue, the answer is "eat until you're full!" And by 'full' I don't mean the old idea, that you've heard repeatedly of being 'moderately full.' I mean, seriously...do you even know what it feels like to be moderately full?... Because I don't!

A more accurate way to think of being 'full' is to think in terms of satiety. Satiety is a way of expressing the state of being physically nourished and satisfied. We all know that feeling. It's the feeling we have when we say, "I'm done" and push the plate away from us. Unfortunately, many of us have been shamed into thinking that it is a 'bad' state to get to. However, the human body has evolved to go out, find food, and then, when it is found, to eat abundantly.

That's why it works so well to eat substantial, real-food meals until we're satisfied, and then go for a period without eating. It's also one of the reasons why periods of fasting are not only normal (in a biological and evolutionary sense) but can also be beneficial *for some people*, especially those who tend to overeat.

A modular approach to meal planning

Modular meal planning is a method for planning and preparing meals that align with your health and performance goals, eliminating the need to count calories. Now, that doesn't mean that counting calories, macros, or tracking isn't valuable; they certainly can be.

However, for much of our time, overly prescriptive plans that dictate exactly how much of a food, macro, or calorie we should consume typically don't work over the long term. They don't provide the same surety that having a good idea of what a meal should look like in your mind's eye offers, especially if you haven't learned to prepare meals *without* using a strict plan.

Why a 'modular' approach?

A modular approach to meal planning helps you understand the components of a well-balanced meal and provides a visual representation to help you create (or purchase) healthy meals at any time and from anywhere.

Nutritional priorities

The general structure for modular meal planning suggests that protein, vegetables, and healthy fats are essential components of a meal and should be prioritised.

Allocating protein first, then vegetables, and finally healthy fats helps ensure that essential amino acids, vitamins, minerals, and essential fatty acids (especially omega-3 fats) are present in the meal.

What about carbohydrate?

As mentioned earlier, carbohydrate-rich foods can be added after other nutrients if you find that you are still hungry or not satisfied. This way, you'll be allocating carbohydrates (which are used almost exclusively for fuel) according to your activity requirements. Your activity levels will drive a greater demand for fuel, which in turn will lead to increased hunger.

Suppose you have sufficient amounts of vegetables, healthy fats, and especially protein in your diet. In that case, this level of hunger should be appropriate to your overall energy requirements, a concept we refer to as 'autoregulation of energy intake'.

So, if, after having your protein, vegetables, and healthy fats, you're still consistently hungry, think about adding some quality carbohydrate to your diet and modify that amount up or down according to your activity and hunger levels (and over time, your body fat level) to find your best balance point.

This is a **Carb-Appropriate** way to find your tolerance and requirement for higher-carb foods and thus eliminates the need to define yourself as either 'low-carb' or 'high-carb'. See an example of how this might work below:

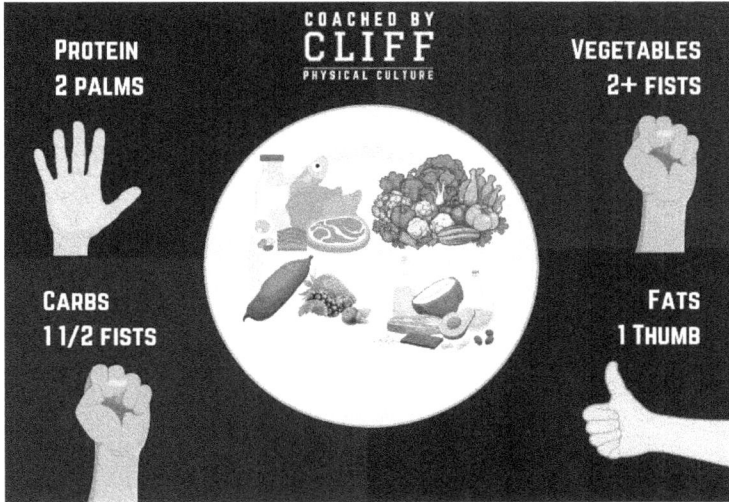

PROTEIN
2 PALMS

COACHED BY
CLIFF
PHYSICAL CULTURE

VEGETABLES
2+ FISTS

CARBS
1 1/2 FISTS

FATS
1 THUMB

To track or not to track?

Tracking calories and macros is a common yet controversial practice. Some believe that tracking your calories and macros closely is the only way to achieve optimal results. In contrast, others suggest that this approach can lead to disordered eating and poorer long-term adherence.

Self-monitoring with mobile-based apps is associated with significant weight loss (of around 2.5 kg over 6 months),[62] and anecdotally, when rapid changes in body composition are desired, tracking results in more consistent results than other approaches.

However, there is also an association between tracking behaviours and disordered eating.[63] In this study, participants who used tracking were also more likely to have higher levels of diet concern and dietary restraint. While this could be an example of *reverse causation* (i.e., those who had latent patterns of disordered eating are more likely to be more inflexible around their eating and more likely to track calories), it's also possible that there are people for whom tracking could push them into disordered eating.

So, is tracking good or bad?

It's neither really. Tracking is a tool that is usually best used for short periods when you have a distinct goal or if you need to 'check in' with yourself. It helps you evaluate your eating to see whether you are meeting your macronutrient targets or are inadvertently over- or undereating.

I track my progress if I want to lose fat rapidly, and I also track for a week or two a year to ensure that I'm hitting my protein targets (which I commonly fail to do). Suffice to say, if you have a tendency towards disordered eating or you find that when tracking, you become excessively rigid or it drives any negative feelings of self-worth, guilt, shame, or anxiety, then forego tracking for other methods.

Autoregulation: Nutrition on autopilot

Autoregulation typically refers to methods used in training to self-adjust training loads or volumes to meet the physical and mental capacity of the athlete within a training session. In nutrition, I began using this term many years ago to describe the ability to eat an appropriate number of calories and be replete in both macro and micronutrients without having to track them. In a nutshell, it describes methods that allow you to eat the right amount without realising you're doing it.

Autoregulation tactics in depth

Protein

Protein is commonly referred to as the most satiating nutrient. While I think it's cavalier to attribute magical properties to any singular nutrient when eating combined, balanced meals is a whole different beast, the evidence does demonstrate that increased protein increases thermogenesis and satiety compared to diets of lower protein content and that high-protein intakes reduce subsequent energy intake.[64]

In a survival setting, we would be inclined to eat what was available to supply the necessary amino acids, even if those foods were not especially high in protein. In other words, having a little is better than going without. *Protein leverage theory* is based on the idea that we will continue to eat (what is readily available) until we have achieved amino acid sufficiency. In one of the few studies directly examining the effects of a high-protein (vs. low-protein) meal, a higher-protein breakfast led to greater feelings of fullness and reduced cravings for both savoury and sweet foods.[65] So, by optimising your protein intake, you will be less likely to overeat.

Fasting

Fasting has become a cause célèbre in the fields of health and nutrition in recent years. Like many issues in nutrition, it is incredibly polarising, with some claiming extraordinary benefits bordering on the magical and others claiming conversely that it results in hormone dysfunction, disordered eating, and should not be done, especially by women. And, like other nutrition-related issues, the truth is likely to be somewhere in the middle.

Overall, the reviews of studies conducted so far indicate that fasting offers a range of health benefits,[67,68] and that much of this benefit stems from energy restriction. By reducing the 'feeding window' available, people tend to eat less overall because, even if they 'overeat' during their non-fasting times, they do not consume more than they would have if not fasting.

It has been observed in randomised controlled trials that fasting does not result in increased calorie intake during the non-fasting times.[66]

So, fasting is an effective way to achieve calorie restriction, but it may also offer additional benefits by encouraging secondary processes, such as reduced insulin-like growth factor (IGF-1), a hormone that, while beneficial to growth and repair, is also implicated in the development of cancer when produced in excess.

Fasting also increases autophagy and apoptosis (self-destruction and immune destruction of dysfunctional cells and tissues),[67] reduces monocyte-driven inflammation and may offer additional benefits beyond simply restricting energy intake.[68] However, while advocates for fasting point to concepts like autophagy, mitophagy, and reduction in monocyte-driven inflammation as (magical!) primary reasons for the results seen from fasting, almost all the benefits result from energy restriction.

So, in a paradigm in which we want to (as much as possible) ensure energy *autoregulation,* fasting can be an appropriate way of eating for those who habitually overeat. On the other hand, it's highly likely that a significant minority of people habitually undereat, leading to effects on training and performance, mood, mental health, and other outcomes (like increased pain). For these people, fasting is not optimal.

Therefore, most people should not fast, or at least not fast aggressively or habitually. People for whom this may be true include not only habitual under-eaters, under-eaters with Gilbert's syndrome, uncontrolled or poorly controlled diabetics who aren't being monitored by a suitably qualified practitioner, or those seeking to gain substantial amounts of muscle and failing to do so.

For those who want to try fasting, there are many different styles available, and much discussion about what is considered the 'best' way to fast. However, there is no single best fasting method. What works for an individual is determined by their physiology and behaviours within their unique psychosocial environment.

The major points of confusion are commonly:

1. How long should I fast?
2. When should I fast? (Particularly, should I fast in the morning or evening?)

How long should I fast?

The answer to the first question is parsimonious. Fast for as long as you need to... Another way to conceptualise this is to think about how long you need to eat or how many meals you can eat to maintain a healthy body weight (for you). If eating the standard three meals per day makes it difficult for you to maintain your body weight, you may want to consider reducing to two meals or a shorter feeding window. If, on the other hand, you are losing weight and you don't want to, you might consider a shorter fasting window or adding a meal or two to your day.

Of course, all of this is predicated on the understanding that you are eating a diet that is based on natural, unrefined foods (to at least 80% of your overall nutrition), and if that's not the case, then THAT is the first step!

When should I fast?

The debate rages as to whether you should fast early (e.g., miss breakfast) or late (i.e., have an early dinner or miss dinner), or something in between!

While different studies and expert opinions will provide evidence for either style, the key is *what you can stick to.* Because there is likely to be a slight difference between these styles over the longer term, it is best to choose a style that suits your unique situation to achieve optimal results.

 The easiest way to evaluate this is to ask yourself the simple question: *Am I hungry when I wake up in the morning?*

If the answer is yes, then eat breakfast! Then, either skip lunch (12:12 fasting) and have your next meal at dinner or after work or have lunch and an early dinner to accommodate the fasting window you want (i.e., 12, 14, 16, or more hours of fasting).

If, on the other hand, you aren't hungry in the morning, there is no good reason to force yourself to eat. Omitting breakfast and then resuming eating either late in the morning, for lunch, late in the afternoon, or even at night, are all good strategies depending on the individual. One of the primary considerations again is to a) make sure you are still eating a healthy diet containing plenty of protein and veggies, and b) make sure that you are taking in enough energy (and macros and micros) to thrive over the longer term.

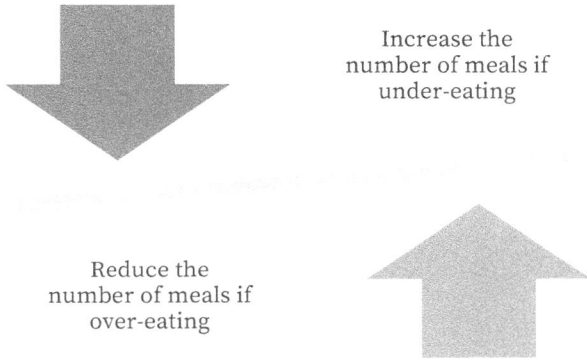

Increase the
number of meals if
under-eating

Reduce the
number of meals if
over-eating

Vegetables

Vegetables provide 'bulk' to the diet. Yes, they also offer additional essential vitamins and minerals and secondary nutrients that help to improve and modulate our total antioxidant capacity, along with gut-healthy fibre and resistant starches that might indirectly also improve satiety by helping to modulate the gut microbiome and via the production of cool short-chain fatty acids (with a host of health benefits). They also help to fill us up. This is due to the two-fold nature of what we consider satiety and satisfaction. The first part of this, and the most discussed, is the recognition of various nutrient chemicals in food and the chemical responses to them (such as modulation of ghrelin and leptin, our key regulators of satiety).

The other aspect, less commonly discussed, is the issue of 'bulk' and how the volume of food provides another stimulus for satiety, resulting from the involvement of the stretch reflex and the enteric nervous system in the gastrointestinal tract.

Carbohydrate

Carbohydrates are (overall) the least satiating nutrient, and so, they are often left out of the discussion of nutritional autoregulation. However, there are important instances in which carbohydrate can improve autoregulation for both habitual over- and under-eaters.

In overeaters, carbohydrates can sometimes improve compliance with a healthy diet by providing an additional source of energy within a meal if the desire for protein, fat, and vegetables has been exhausted. While usually this would be only a limited amount, as the overall desire is to consume more protein-rich and nutrient-dense, high-bulk foods, if one has exhausted their willingness to eat foods of that type, but they haven't eaten enough overall, a case could be made that by excessively restricting carbohydrates, the person might be more likely to rebound overeat.

It's also important to always remember that we eat foods, not 'nutrients', and there are carbohydrate foods that are considered incredibly satiating (such as potatoes). When these and other higher-bulk carbohydrate foods are included and prioritised over lower-satiety (and typically highly refined) carb choices, this can also improve autoregulation in the overeater.

It should be noted, however, that single-food satiety plays a lesser role when considering mixed meals. For example, how often would you eat a potato cooked without anything else, on its own? My guess is not often... Most people are more likely to consume it with butter, sour cream, or fried!

Diets *extremely* high in carbohydrate and based on a foundation of mostly unrefined foods are also as or more satiating as lower-carbohydrate diets previously thought to be the 'best' for satiety.[69] This lends credence to the idea that 'bookend' approaches (either low-carb or very low-fat) offer the best satiety and therefore, autoregulation 'down'.

Of course, the approach that you should take depends on your food preferences and other factors (like how easy it would be to supply protein and essential omega-3 fatty acids in a very-low-fat, high-carb diet). In under-eaters, the case is even clearer. Adding carbohydrate foods to mixed meals that aren't overly restricted in fat content helps increase the overall volume of food and energy consumed.

Fats

Like carbohydrates, fat isn't particularly satiating. However, when combined with protein and vegetables in the desired amounts (according to your goal), we have observed an additive effect. The take-home message is quite simple: supply enough essential fatty acids and preformed long-chain omega-3 fats (DHA and EPA) and ensure that the fat in your diet aligns with your dietary strategy, typically with at least 30% of your calories coming from dietary fat.

Sleep

It is known that sleep duration influences weight gain, as well as the development of overweight and obesity, and the resulting health effects of these conditions.[70-72] This is likely to be due in part to the impact sleep has on autoregulation.

Partial sleep deprivation results in increased energy intake (i.e. you eat more), and people who overeat as a result of sleep deprivation tend to consume more fat and less protein,[73] and have a poorer diet overall,[74] characterised by more snacking and soda use.[75]

This relationship is also bidirectional, with a poorer diet likely to lead to poorer sleep.[74] Conversely, getting adequate sleep is associated with a higher intake of fruits and vegetables.[75]

So, sleep, while being critical to health overall, is also an essential part of being able to stick to a healthy diet and eat an appropriate amount of energy...without even realising you're doing it!

Stress

There is a strong bidirectional relationship between stress, sleep, and food intake. In other words, factors like stress worsen sleep and increase food intake, resulting in weight gain, and conversely, worsened sleep drives poorer food choices, and poor food choices worsen sleep (and obesity is a known risk for sleep disorders).[76]

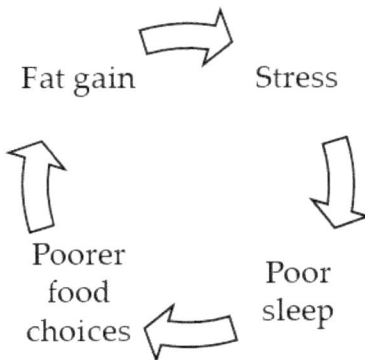

Fat gain → Stress → Poor sleep → Poorer food choices →

Chronic stress promotes a shift to overeating. This contrasts with acute stress, which typically reduces food intake due to the catecholamine stress hormones that act as both stimulants and appetite suppressants. Hyperactivation of stress responses promotes metabolic shifts that encourage fat gain and increase inflammation, which in turn is associated with further fat gain. Additionally, detrimental changes occur in the gut microbiota, which could also contribute to a trend towards adiposity.[77]

Different people may also have differing effects on autoregulation related to stress. Research suggests that in leaner participants (which might include 'hardgainer' types who struggle to gain muscle), stress was more likely to be related to weight loss. In contrast, those with more weight or body fat were more likely to gain weight (however, this effect wasn't seen in women).[78]

Excessive and chronic stress can impede optimal autoregulation, typically favouring weight gain, but also potentially minimise muscle gain and reduce already low energy intakes in chronic under-eaters.

Quantifying nutrition

If you want to fine-tune your nutrition, autoregulation alone may not be enough. You might want to quantify your nutrition for peace of mind or because you're a more analytical person. Still, I don't think it's worth 'over-engineering' your diet. A simple strategy using the following steps is often all that someone requires, unless they are a high-level athlete needing to define their carbohydrate intake more precisely.

- Calculate your energy intake: Aim to be within 10% of this target
- Calculate your minimum desired protein intake: Exceed this target every day
- Leave the fat and carbohydrate intake flexible to meet the energy target above

Calculate energy requirements

In previous books, I **(Cliff)** have included formulas for calorie calculations, but to be honest, nowadays it is easier and more convenient to find an online calculator or use an app like Cronometer or MyFitnessPal to roughly estimate your daily energy requirements. While these are not entirely accurate (nor are any calculations), they provide a starting point from which you can adjust if you are not meeting your muscle gain or fat loss goals (i.e., by increasing or reducing your calorie intake).

Allocate macronutrients

Splitting energy intake into macronutrients requires the application of evidence-based best practices and a healthy dose of common sense, while also considering your specific needs. Rough guidelines are as follows:

Nutrient	Recommended Intake	Adjustments
Protein	More than 1.4-2.2 g/kg/day	Up to 3.1 g/LBM/day if desired, dieting or undereating
Fat	Minimum ~40-60 g per day or ~1 g/kg/LBM	20-80% of calories depending on need

For example, if one is following a lower-carb diet, they might consume 40-80% of calories from fat, moderate carbs might mean 20-40% of calories from carbs, and a high-carb diet might mean less than 30% of calories from carbs.

Note: Athletes typically derive between 20% and 40% of their energy from fat.

What about carbohydrate?

Carbohydrates should account for the remaining energy intake. Still, as stated earlier, if one is meeting their required energy intake and exceeding their minimum protein intake, day-to-day variations in the relative amount of carbs vs fat that one consumes are unlikely to make any appreciable difference. The allocation of fat or carbohydrate in meals and the diet overall becomes more a function of dietary sustainability (how easily you can stick to a healthy diet) than how effective the diet will be per se.

Note: For optimal sporting performance, carbohydrate is suggested to be equal to or greater than 5 g/kg/day, and in extreme sporting durations, up to 12 g/kg/day.

Supplements

We hear repeatedly from nutrition experts that supplements are unnecessary and that 'all you need to do is eat a good diet and you'll get all that you need.' While this is technically correct, we need to consider that a) many of us won't eat well enough to be replete in all essential nutrients consistently, and b) having higher than 'normal' intakes of some nutrients (e.g., protein) is beneficial if we want not just to survive but thrive and live to our fullest potential. Not to mention that while we are getting our diets in order, we might also benefit from some nutritional support.

On the other hand, in the supplement industry, there are numerous quacks and snake-oil products alongside legitimate supplements that have been well-proven to work. This leads inevitably to confusion. With all the hyped products that don't work and the plethora of effective ones, it can be challenging to determine which supplements to use.

We can make sense of supplementation by looking at it as a 'hierarchy of needs' like Maslow's hierarchy of human social needs. The 'base' of this hierarchy is food, and this is where this model and I agree with the 'just eat a healthy diet' crowd. The more essential and beneficial secondary nutrients that your base diet can provide, the better.

Next, it is prudent to use what I call 'food-like supplements' to provide 'nutritional insurance' to your diet. The first of these is a good multinutrient providing at least recommended daily amounts of all the essential vitamins and minerals (except perhaps iron due to the relatively high incidence of sub-clinical iron overload) and preferably, also secondary nutrients from wholefoods to provide a 'matrix' of synergistic nutrients beneficial to health. Next up are other food-like supplements that help mitigate common nutrient deficiencies, especially fish oil. Fourthly, we can begin to apply some specific nutrients based on our needs, for example, magnesium and zinc before bed if we are having trouble sleeping and/or if food analysis or blood testing shows that we are low in these nutrients, and vitamin D if we don't get enough sun, live in an area where sun exposure is low (especially in winter) and/or if we have an immune-related disorder in which vitamin D is likely to be beneficial.

For this tier of supplementation, it is advisable to consult a qualified and registered dietitian or clinical nutritionist, as their recommendations will be tailored to your specific needs, diet, lifestyle, and individual test results. Finally, some ergogenic and specific application supplements round out the hierarchy. These would be considered optional but might give appreciable benefits. There are also a few things to experiment with for a bit of fun.

Creatine is a good example of an evidence-based, proven ergogenic supplement, the undisputed king of supplements.

HPN HIERARCHY OF SUPPLEMENTATION

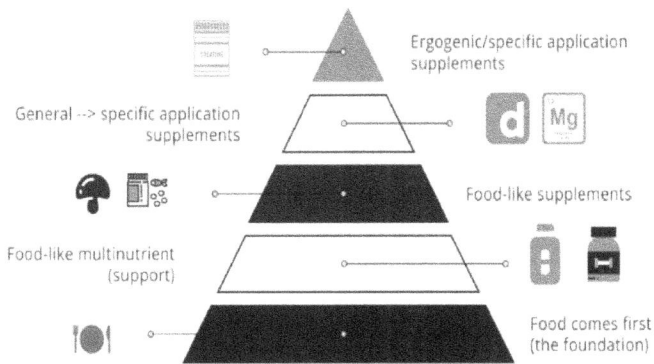

Cliff's key nutrition tactic

There are no 'rules' for nutrition; there's just what works. Even the overarching strategies previously mentioned are not rules that you *must* follow. They are suggestions that work for most people, most of the time. Similarly, these are tactics that work well for me (and many of my clients) to make healthy and adequate nutrition easier.

Two meals & two shakes per day

One of the benefits of focusing on meals rather than snacks is that it frees you from excessive meal preparation. Even just the thought of prepping three meals and three snacks every day stresses me out! Sure, I used to do it back in the '90s. Like many others into strength and physique sports, I carried around a cooler with meals and shakes to get me through the day, lest I go a few hours without protein and waste away to pencil-neck status!

We subsequently realised that this wasn't necessary to grow and maintain muscle (and strength), and this realisation freed us from the clock, making life a lot simpler.

I became a competitive strength athlete at around the same time as my clinical practice was really taking off. I had a dual focus back in those days: strength coaching & personal training, and nutrition. I would wake up at around 4.30 am, do a little writing, then head into the gym to train my first client at 6 am, train clients through the morning, then head back after lunch to my clinic, see clients for nutrition in the afternoon, and then head up to the Millennium Institute to train for a few hours. After that, I'd get home, make dinner, and crash out!

There wasn't a lot of spare time. So, I developed the pattern that I still (mostly) follow all these years later, and which incidentally has been used by many of my high-performing athlete clients.

I mix up 2-3 smoothie 'meals' in the morning (or the night before) so that I have those meals ready-to-go. At night, my partner, Bella, and I make dinner (in fairness, she does most of the cooking nowadays!) and prepare enough for lunch the following day or for several subsequent days. This way, we can be assured of getting in the energy, protein, and essential nutrients we require with a minimum of fuss and prep time.

So, my current routine looks something like this:

- On waking: 2 glasses of water, multinutrient drink with egg white protein, a Tbsp of collagen, a Greens/Multi, & fish oil
- Training

- After training: Smoothie #1
- Lunch: Meal (leftovers from previous night)
- After work (around 3-4 pm): Smoothie #2
- Dinner: Meal

Meals are simple, yet delicious, and are made up of meat, fish, chicken, or occasionally a vegetarian meal based on beans, lentils, tofu, or tempeh, along with plenty of vegetables, healthy fats (typically flax or olive oil as the base for dressings) and carbohydrate depending on our current goals (less if training less or losing fat, more if training more and/or in a hypertrophy phase). Carbs are typically from Kūmara (sweet potato), potato, or rice.

Smoothies follow the general structure of:

1. Protein powder (use whey, pea protein isolate, egg white, or beef hydrolysate protein depending on tolerance and personal preference)
2. Healthy fats to the desired amount (flax oil, fish oil, MCT oil, olive oil, etc.)
3. Creatine (and perhaps some other clever nutrients like nicotinamide riboside, n-acetylcysteine, or various mushroom extracts)
4. Berries and/or tropical fruit
5. Sometimes I add vegetables if I'm not getting enough at my other meals

Sometimes, I'll also add collagen powder, green powder, mushroom powder, or extracts, or other supplements that I'm using for a specific outcome.

Summary

- **Make two shakes in the morning**
- **Consume one in the morning and one in the afternoon**
- **Make too much at dinner so that you have a quality meal for the following day's lunch**

11

MODIFICATIONS

What if you want to lose fat, or gain muscle, or achieve a specific health or performance outcome? Modifications are necessary to ensure you are reaching the goals that matter to you and can adjust your diet and lifestyle as those goals evolve and shift over time.

Maximum fat loss

If your goal is maximal fat loss, or if your tests from earlier in the book (especially the waist-to-height ratio) indicate that you should lose some body fat, you may need to make a few modifications to your plan. However, you might not need to either!

For many people, simply following an intelligent strength training plan, with some additional residual activity (like a daily work and/or some 'play' activities) and taking an autoregulation approach to nutrition will be all they need. For some, though, a slightly more aggressive approach, at least for a time, might be necessary.

Now, it bears saying that it is neither 'impossible' to lose fat after 40 nor is 'middle-aged spread' inevitable. However, there is some degree of resistance to fat loss, making it more challenging to reduce body fat and maintain a lower body fat percentage as we age.

This inevitably leads to the question: *How lean is lean enough?*

The simple answer is that if you are regularly engaged in strength training and residual activity, and eat a diet mainly based on unrefined foods that is replete in all the essential nutrients and high in secondary nutrients beneficial to health, then you're likely to be as lean as you need to be and this should be indicated by a waist-height ratio of less than 0.5 (in other words, your waist circumference is no more than ½ of your height).

You might want to be leaner for aesthetic reasons or because you want to maintain a lower body weight for weight-restricted sports, both of which are good, but (depending on how lean you want to be), will require more diligence with your nutrition and lifestyle. There will inevitably be diminishing returns, wherein the pursuit of leanness becomes counterproductive to health, happiness, or performance.

To take a broad and healthy 'autoregulation' approach to the next level for fat loss, people typically follow one of two strategies: one that is less time- and energy-consuming but also less quantifiable, and the other more rigid but far more quantifiable. These are exclusionary and tracking approaches.

Exclusion approach

In an exclusion approach to fat loss, people typically exclude or drastically reduce food groups or types of nutrients, most commonly carbohydrates. By doing so, they can reduce overall energy intake, prioritise protein (which has a lesser effect on fat gain), and reduce hyperpalatable 'trigger' foods that drive higher food (and therefore energy) intake.

Does this mean that carbohydrates are bad or that you can't lose fat on a higher-carb diet?

Nope, not in the slightest, it's just that many people find that they can (at least for a time) stick to a diet that removes many of the foods that they typically overeat and that drive them to want to eat more. While there is a lot of debate about whether a low-carb diet is in fact superior to a low-fat (and higher-carb) diet for fat loss, overall, the evidence points to there being little difference between otherwise healthy diets for fat loss and health outcomes over the long term if they are equivalent in energy (calories).

In an exclusionary approach, we aim to find a straightforward way to reduce energy intake by avoiding specific foods. In other words, this is a way, not the only way.

Strategy 1. A gradual restriction of higher-carbohydrate foods

Why restriction?

- Abstinence is often easier than moderation
- Allows for a simple method of elimination diet (for allergies and intolerances)
- Allows for this elimination in an easily integrated fashion and reduces potential metabolic or digestive disruptors.

Abstinence is easier than moderation

There is a lack of research on the effects of moderation vs. abstinence on diet outcomes. However, clinical experience suggests that it is a simpler 'mind-set' for people to consider one, clear elimination strategy at a time (in which they avoid a specific food entirely), rather than having to quantify and then reduce food types or particular macronutrients and count calories.

Steps along the 'stepwise' approach serve to reduce the total glycaemic load in the diet. Because lower-carb diets have demonstrated greater satiety, improved compliance, and better autoregulation, they offer a more effective path to fat loss than starving oneself.

Benefits for identifying allergies and intolerances

Elimination diets are also a real-life test of food intolerances. In fact, many medical texts prioritise this type of elimination testing as one of the few credible ways to determine intolerances. This is not the primary purpose of the stepwise approach. Still, if, when following a gradual restriction of carbohydrate, you notice reduced symptoms of food intolerance (i.e., improved energy and wellbeing, reduced gastrointestinal symptoms, enhanced cognitive performance and reduced skin conditions and nasal congestion), you can better identify food types to which you are intolerant.

Strategy 2. A drastic reduction in carbohydrate foods with a longer-term 'back off'

In this approach, one would start at the other end of the 'staircase' in the image above, eliminating most obligate carbohydrate foods until the desired results are achieved. Then, carbohydrate foods can be reintroduced (to a level of tolerance) for either maintenance or when transitioning into a phase of greater muscle and strength gain.

Limitations of carb-restriction

While restricting carbohydrates is a common and effective approach for fat loss, many people will benefit more from a higher-carb, lower-fat approach. I know that comes as a shock to the keto-zealots, and while the evidence isn't clear-cut, what we do see in the research and in nutrition practice bears this out.

Who benefits most from higher-carb and lower-carb diets?

Preliminary randomised controlled trials that have been performed show that people with *relative* insulin resistance (IR) achieve greater fat loss from a low-carbohydrate diet, while those who are more insulin sensitive (IS) get better results from a higher-carbohydrate diet.[79-83]

Taken on balance, these results suggest that individuals who are more insulin resistant and those with metabolic syndrome (prediabetes) may achieve better results from low-carb diets. Conversely, those who are insulin-sensitive may achieve better results for weight loss and fat loss, as well as improvements in cardiometabolic risk markers, from higher-carb and lower-fat diets. However, it is also important to remember that on these energy-restricted diets, people achieved weight loss irrespective of the diet allocation. This reinforces that a relative energy deficit (i.e., expending more energy than you consume) is the primary determinant of fat and weight loss.

Do activity and sport affect the type of diet I should be eating?

I've been saying for nearly 30 years that *carbohydrate intake is activity-dependent*. In other words, higher volumes of exercise, and especially higher volumes of repeated higher-intensity bouts of exercise, increase the requirement for carbohydrate due to the glycolytic (carb-burning) nature of that exercise and the limited capacity to store muscle and liver glycogen for use. This general rule applies regardless of whether one is following a low-, moderate-, or high-carbohydrate baseline diet.

When to consider *increasing* carbohydrate intake

- If you are increasing the volume of glycolytic activity (i.e., adding sessions of conditioning-style workouts), especially if the athlete is unable to achieve optimal performance.

- If sleep quality decreases, menstrual irregularities appear, anxiety levels increase or unwanted symptoms occur (i.e., hair loss, keto-rash), and this is suspected to be due to energy deficit.
  Note: This may be more prevalent in females, primarily due to their higher hormonal sensitivity compared to males, to sudden changes in diet or overall energy availability.

- If you prefer (or you can stick to) dietary strategies with a greater carbohydrate intake.

- If you are consistently undereating

Specific to the strength-training over-40 athlete:

- When trying to gain substantial amounts of mass or muscle

Specific to over-40 athletes who engage in endurance training:

- To support longer sessions that include >45 minutes of higher intensity glycolytic work (i.e., intervals, hill climbs, sprints).
- During competition periods

- If not gaining muscle during a hypertrophy phase of training (assuming sufficient protein and energy intake)

In any of the above conditions, small increments of carbohydrate (i.e., ½ a fist-sized portion at each meal) can be added until the desired effect is achieved, such as improving top-end performance or eliminating symptoms or side effects.

When to consider *reducing* carbohydrate intake

- If you are consistently overeating (also consider if your current protein and vegetable intake is adequate)

- If you need to reduce excess and unwanted body fat AND you adhere better to a lower-carbohydrate approach

- If your volume of total activity and especially highly glycolytic activity is decreasing

- If you do not like or adhere well to higher-carbohydrate intakes

- If a lower carbohydrate approach is preferred for the management of co-existing metabolic (i.e., type 1 or 2 diabetes) or neurological conditions. *Note: Please consult with a qualified and registered nutrition professional for guidance.*

It should be noted that even athletes who are lower-carb can benefit from increased carbohydrate during events, higher-volume training phases, and peri-training carbohydrate nutrition.

These can still be consistent with a low-carb approach if that works best for you on a day-to-day basis.

Muscle gain

Carbohydrate is anabolic…

So, for muscle gain, it is typically (although not always) preferable to have a moderate or higher carbohydrate intake. In any event, for most people, muscle mass increases benefit from an increased carbohydrate and energy surplus (taking in more than you expend) and sufficient protein (usually at least 1.6 g of protein per kg of body weight per day).

Good food, bad foods…

Whenever one talks or writes about health and strength, there will be inevitable questions about which foods are 'good' and 'bad'. So, let's dispel that myth right now.

There are no good or bad foods *per se*. Instead, the overall context of all the foods you eat, collectively known as your diet, is the key to health.

This means that we can enjoy treats and discretionary foods while still pursuing and achieving health and happiness.

Of course, if we overdo certain foods, we will experience poorer health outcomes for two primary reasons. Firstly, ultra-processed foods can 'crowd out' more nutrient-dense options, leaving us lacking in essential micronutrients that the body needs to fulfil all of its functions (including, but not limited to, immunity, fat loss, muscle gain, mood, and cognition) and secondly, hyperpalatable foods – typically those that are ultra-processed and higher in sugar, or sugar or other highly processed carbohydrate in combination with fat, generally are not as satiating as foods that are closer to their whole state. This leads to overeating, which is why sugar-sweetened beverages and convenience foods are associated with obesity and chronic diseases like diabetes and cardiovascular disease.

How to have your cake and eat it!

Traversing the 'treat food' minefield can be one of the most challenging aspects of changing one's health status. However, we can find strategies within our health that allow us to enjoy the foods we love while also achieving our health goals.

Key concept: Freedom within structure

I (Cliff) talk a lot with my clients about the idea of *freedom within structure*. As humans, we crave freedom and rebel against constraint. This has led to various movements of food freedom within the nutrition world. Unfortunately, simply 'eating intuitively' seldom results in positive physical health outcomes, although it is beneficial to one's mindset and mental health.

On the other hand, rigid and inflexible approaches to nutrition are also unsuitable and typically lead to rebound eating and the phenomenon of 'yo-yo dieting'.

We can find some pragmatic middle ground, though. Freedom within structure involves finding tactics that you can apply that allow you to eat healthy, nourishing foods most of the time while allowing for discretionary foods that you eat more for their taste and psychosocial benefits than beneficial effects on your physiology.

Some of the tactics I use with clients are as follows.

Change your food environment

The relative availability of generally 'healthy' and discretionary foods is a critical, yet underappreciated factor in becoming and staying healthy.

We tend to think about our 'control' of what we eat as a 'top-down' process in which we force ourselves to change the way we act. And while willpower and intention are critical to success, they are also limited. When our environment pushes us to do things we don't intend, it can be hard to do the right thing!

Of course, our food environment depends on social, economic, geographical, cultural, and personal factors, all of which are interrelated. However, we can still do our best to change our in-home food environment to one that is conducive to achieving our goals.

The research on proximity to poorer quality foods is enlightening. For example, proximity to fast-food outlets is associated with increased body mass,[84] and childhood obesity and weight gain.[85-87] Living in a 'food desert' or 'food swamp'[i] is significantly associated with a higher body mass,[88] obesity and diabetes.[89]

Both food insecurity and less cooking at home are associated with poorer diet quality,[90-92] but conversely, cooking at home is associated with improved diet quality.[93]

---

[i] A 'food desert' is an area lacking adequate availability of fresh, whole foods. A 'food swamp' is similar but combines a lack of fresh, whole foods with high availability of fast foods and convenience options.

Choose to have healthy, nourishing foods in the home

The home food environment is known to improve dietary quality.[94] For example, research has demonstrated that when parents have a less positive attitude towards junk food and sugar-sweetened beverages, and when these are limited in availability at home, adolescents displayed more autonomous restriction of these foods.[95] Mexican adolescents also reported that they were more likely to consume sugar-sweetened beverages when these were in the home.[96]

Similarly (and surprisingly), parental pressure to eat fruit was not associated with the likelihood of fruit consumption by children, but greater availability was.[97] Children of parents with lower vegetable consumption were 59% less likely to eat vegetables daily. Additionally, watching television for more than one hour per day was associated with a drastic reduction in vegetable intake and a doubled likelihood of consuming sweets or sugar-sweetened beverages at least once per week.[97]

The home environment also seems to influence behaviours that occur autonomously and away from home. In research from England on children aged 6-7 years, higher sugar intakes at home led to a preference for higher sugar foods at lunch.[98]

While much of this research focuses on children, it illustrates that if certain foods are more readily available, we are more likely to eat them. Once we develop a pattern of eating certain things, we continue to consume more of them!

The take-home message is to have almost entirely healthy, whole foods in the home. This doesn't mean you can't have treats; it's just that a better strategy is to make eating them intentional, not a default position when you are tired or stressed.

Be intentional with your treats

Intentionality is a key trait of people who develop prodigious health and strength. But this doesn't mean that you need to be overly rigid with your intentions either. It simply means that there should be some structure or plan for how you will approach 'treat' foods.

For example, my partner and I eat mostly 'healthily' (and I recognise the flaws in that word!) most of the week. Still, on Friday night, we will either go out to dinner (more rarely since we have had kids!) or order takeout, AND we'll have some chocolate, cookies, or some other sweet treat after dinner.

In effect, we 'take the brakes off' for the night. This inevitably bleeds over to the following night, especially if we have leftovers, but the daytime meals are reasonably consistent with what we do during the week (because daytime eating becomes so habitual over time), and by Sunday, everything is back on track.

This strategy is effective for us, but it's not by any means the only one. We also occasionally have treats at other times, and we don't beat ourselves up about it because, on balance, we're achieving our goals.

Moderation vs abstinence

Different approaches work for other people. Some people tend towards an 'abstinence' approach where they achieve their goals most effectively by practically eliminating any trigger foods that lead them to overeat (apart from occasional, intentional treats). In contrast, others do better with a moderation approach, allowing themselves small amounts of discretionary foods more frequently.

I once had a client who rang me up in tears. They were absolutely at their wits' end because they (in their words) 'could not quit chocolate!' When we explored this, it turned out that they were only having four squares of dark chocolate after dinner every night. The thing is, they lost body fat, gained muscle, improved health markers, and achieved their athletic goals. So, I told them

175

not to stress about it at all and to keep eating that (tiny!) amount of chocolate, even if it was every day.

The client, influenced by the adverse effects of media-driven diet culture, developed the idea that they should eliminate all chocolate. In reality, chocolate was a perfect moderator, and their diet and lifestyle overall were entirely conducive to achieving their goals.

Quantifying 'treats'

There is no set number or amount of discretionary foods that anyone should eat. I have known people who avoid them entirely, and others who thrive despite having relatively large amounts of cookies or chocolate every night. It depends on your physiology, your goals, and your psychoemotional and psychosocial milieu.

However, I do use a simple metric myself, especially when I need to 'reset' and focus on my health if I feel that it's beginning to drift.

The 20-10-5 method

This method is one that I have used with clients and myself with great success. It refers to the percentage of your meals that can be 'free' or 'treat' meals.

When I'm in a maintenance phase, am low on stress, replete with nutrients and sleep, and training well, I can typically 'get away with' about 20% of my week's meals being freer. So, as I eat around five meals per day, this equates to around seven meals per week.

If I'm looking to lean up or optimise my health, I might cut back to around 10% of freer meals, or 3-4 meals per week. And when I really want to 'dial in', especially if I'm losing a little body fat to make a lower weight class in weightlifting or BJJ (or for the beach!) I might drop that to 5%, or two 'treat' meals per week.

Change the meals that don't matter

Suffice to say that you don't need to quantify at all if you don't want to. Just make sure that all the meals that don't matter for social or other enjoyment are healthy ones.

Now, of course, healthy meals are also delicious, and so we shouldn't drift into the mindset that healthy = unpalatable and unhealthy = tasty.

What I mean, though, is that many of the meals that you eat during that day don't have the same social or emotional 'weight' as those you enjoy with friends, with your partner, at those special moments like relaxing in front of a movie on a Friday night.

The meals we eat during the workday, when we're getting ready for work, or when we get home from work, do not need to be 'treats', but they can be delicious. Suppose we have created a good food environment at home, with ample amounts of quality proteins, carbs, healthy fats, and vegetables. In that case, we can prepare a robust and nutritious meal as easily as one that isn't as healthy. It will likely be even more delicious.

Alcohol

Lately, earlier research linking alcohol to health benefits has come under fire. This has led many to say that there is *no safe intake* of it. However, this 'no safe dose' messaging is not what the data say!

While there isn't any health benefit from drinking alcohol, it is likely, based on the available evidence, that light drinking is not associated with early death.

A now much-cited 2023 meta-analysis found no significant effect on overall mortality (after adjustment) for up to 44 g of alcohol per day (~4 standard drinks) for men and 25 g for women (2 ½ standard drinks).[99] However, lower intakes than this *are* likely to increase the risk for many cancers, especially in women.[100–102]

It is also clear that heavy drinking is detrimental socially, putting one at much greater risk of accidents and violence. There are also possible risks of addiction and abuse arising from otherwise healthy use, and so, a common-sense recommendation is that **if you don't currently drink, there is no good reason to start.**

On the other hand, if you do drink, it is prudent for health to keep your intake down to under seven drinks per week, with no more than two drinks per day and 'alcohol-free' days each week.

Common-sense tactics

If you currently drink, limit your intake by only buying enough for the week. For example, if you drink beer and are male, you could buy no more than a 6-pack per week and preferably buy light beer, which would further reduce your alcohol intake. If you finish them, that's it, no more for that week. If you don't, roll them over to the following week *and don't restock until they are gone.*

If you drink wine, buying only one bottle of wine per week is a great start.

Also consider the following:

- Have alcohol-free (preferably sugar-free) options available.
- Drink a glass of water between drinks.
- Limit drinks to a maximum of 2-3 on any given day.

If you find yourself consistently drinking more than what is recommended for health, consider seeing a registered mental health practitioner who can help you understand your reasons for drinking and work with you to discover strategies and tactics to reduce or stop your drinking. You can also reflect and do some self-work on why you drink to excess and begin a process of self-discovery.

Coffee

Alternative health practitioners routinely single out coffee as something to be avoided. However, the evidence consistently shows positive effects on a range of health outcomes and on overall mortality from moderate coffee intakes up to ~4 per day.[103,104]

Coffee (or more specifically caffeine) is also an ergogenic (performance-enhancing) substance, providing both physical[105-110] and mental performance and mood benefits,[111-113] and it can help to facilitate fat loss by increasing fat oxidation and reducing appetite (albeit by a small amount).[114-116]

More recently, many have claimed that caffeine increases cortisol levels and is 'bad' for stress and for hormonal regulation, especially in women. However, that claim fails to take into account the *dose* commonly used in research, which is typically 3-6+ mg of caffeine per kg of body weight. For example, caffeine ingestion increases cortisol levels at doses of ≥6 mg/kg.[117,118] Taking 800 mg of caffeine one hour before resistance exercise resulted in a significant increase in cortisol, but 0, 200, and 400 mg did not.[119]

To put that in perspective, up to four cups of strong coffee taken in one sitting did not significantly increase cortisol! So, there is little risk with daily, habitual doses of caffeine.

Take-home message: If you enjoy coffee, then keep on enjoying it! However, if you are struggling with sleep, or you find that you get nervous, anxious, 'jittery', or your mood is depressed after drinking coffee, then consider reducing or removing it.

I typically advise clients to limit their intake to less than 3 mg of caffeine per kilogram of body weight per day, taken in the morning. Clinical experience suggests that this is a tolerable and effective dose for most people, without any adverse effects. For me, this equates to ~270 mg of caffeine per day, or up to three strong cups of coffee.

12

SLEEP

The importance of sleep has been an under-recognised piece of the health puzzle. It wasn't ignored entirely, but the conversation primarily revolved around diet and exercise. Now, we are increasingly beginning to see the enormous role that healthy sleeping patterns play in our overall health and performance. Consequently, a large and growing body of research investigates the roles that sleep plays in contributing to health, as well as the ways it helps improve our health and performance.

What happens when we sleep?

When we sleep, our body reduces sensory and muscle activity, and our consciousness enters an altered state. During sleep, we progress through several distinct phases. These are broadly categorised as rapid eye movement (REM) and non-REM sleep.

During sleep, due to the reduced overall activity, the body can accelerate its recovery by building tissue and restoring immune and hormone functions. It has also recently been discovered that sleep plays a crucial role in removing toxins produced by normal day-to-day functioning from the brain. These metabolites are not removed during the day, but when we sleep, they are rhythmically 'washed' from the brain and central nervous system by the *glymphatic* (glial + lymphatic) system. Much of the body's rebuilding, repair, and waste removal occurs during REM sleep.

The cycles of sleep

Within minutes, we enter stage one sleep, characterised by alpha and theta brain waves. After several minutes of light sleep, we enter stage two. This stage is characterised by bursts of neural activity.

Deep sleep (also called *slow-wave sleep*) involves stages three and four. In these stages, muscle activity is inhibited, and it is harder to awaken. The brain produces more delta waves. In this stage, much of the body's repair occurs; therefore, getting enough deep sleep is critical to health.

About 90 minutes after falling asleep, we enter REM sleep, characterised by rapid, jerking movements of the eyes. In this phase, the brain reactivates (most dreaming occurs during REM sleep). REM sleep plays a key role in learning and memory function, as it allows the brain to process and organise this information.[ii]

Sleep Phases

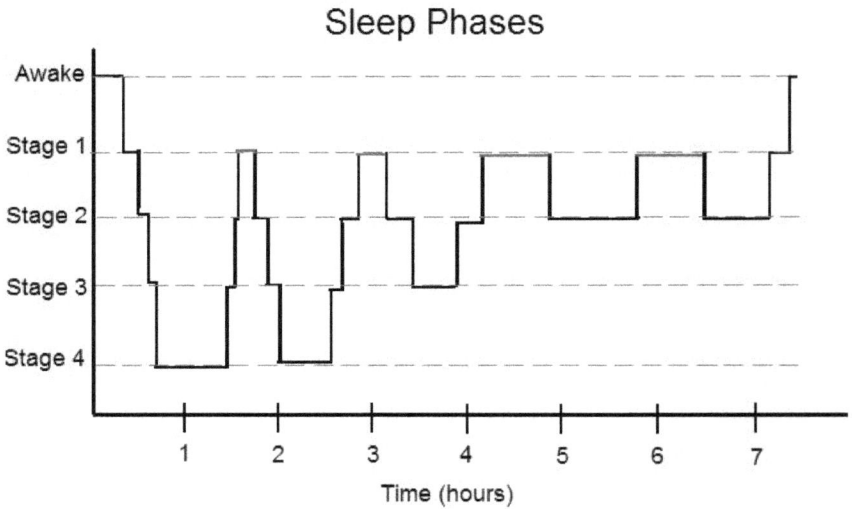

[ii] Kernsters [CC BY-SA (https://creativecommons.org/licenses/by-sa/3.0)]
https://commons.wikimedia.org/wiki/File:Simplified_Sleep_Phases.jpg

How much sleep should we get?

According to the National Sleep Foundation in the US, which convened an expert panel to evaluate optimal sleep times, the recommended amounts of sleep for various ages are[120]:

- 0-3 months: 14-17 hours per night
- 4-11 months: 12-15 hours
- 1-2 years: 11-14 hours
- 3-5 years: 10-13 hours
- 6-13 years: 9-11 hours
- 14-17 years: 8-10 hours
- **18-64 years: 7-9 hours**
- **65+ years: 7-8 hours**

However, the *quality* of sleep is also crucial, with adequate periods of deep sleep and REM sleep. While there is no consensus on exactly how much REM and deep sleep are required for optimal function, deep sleep should account for at least 13% of total sleep duration. In comparison, REM sleep typically accounts for at least 20% of sleep in healthy individuals.[121]

There can also be significant variations between individuals. While most of us perform best within the norms suggested above, variability exists among people, and some thrive on different sleep times and patterns.

The effects of sleep deprivation on health

Both short and excessively long sleep durations (which are often a consequence of disease and disorder) are associated with early death and increased risk of diabetes, metabolic syndrome,[122,123] cardiovascular diseases, and strokes.[124–128]

Poor sleep has also been shown to worsen cognitive abilities, and conversely, better sleep improves the ability to store memories for later retrieval.[129] In cross-sectional studies of sleep duration and cognition, extremes of sleep duration were significantly associated with poorer performance over multiple domains (such as performance, executive function, verbal memory, and working memory).[130] Those with sleep-disordered breathing were 26% more likely to develop cognitive impairment.[131]

Studies also suggest that sleep disturbances can increase the risk of dementia. For example, people with sleep problems have been demonstrated to have a 68% greater likelihood of cognitive impairment or Alzheimer's disease, and approximately 15% of Alzheimer's disease in the population may be attributed to sleep problems.[132] In a meta-analysis of studies including over 69000 participants, individuals with sleep problems had around 55% to 400% greater risk of a range of cognitive challenges, including Alzheimer's disease, cognitive impairment, and preclinical Alzheimer's disease, than people without sleep problems.[132]

On a day-to-day basis, sleep quality, duration of sleep, and sleep latency (the time taken to get to sleep) are known to affect mood,[133] and increase anxiety,[134,135] and depression risk.[136]

A robust connection between sleep disorders and neurodegenerative diseases has also been drawn. For example, in those with a REM sleep disorder (disabling the ability to achieve proper REM sleep), the risk of developing a neurodegenerative disease was 33.5% at five years follow-up, 82.4% at 10.5 years and 96.6% at 14 years, with nearly half of these developing Parkinson's disease.[137]

It is important to note that *correlation does not equal causation.* Illnesses and health conditions can alter sleep patterns (through physical pain and discomfort or mental and emotional anguish). Still, poor sleeping patterns do alter physiological processes that contribute to poor health, and the relationship is bidirectional – sleep can worsen health. Poorer health can also exacerbate sleep issues, leading to a vicious cycle.

Sleep duration influences fat gain and the risk of being overweight and obese.[70] Under-sleeping results in increased energy intake (i.e. you eat more), and when people overeat as a result of sleep deprivation, they tend to eat more fat and less protein,[73] have a poorer diet overall,[74] snack more and drink more soda.[75]

This relationship is bidirectional; a poorer diet leads to poorer sleep, and poorer sleep leads to a poorer diet![74] Conversely, getting adequate sleep is associated with a higher intake of fruits and vegetables.[75]

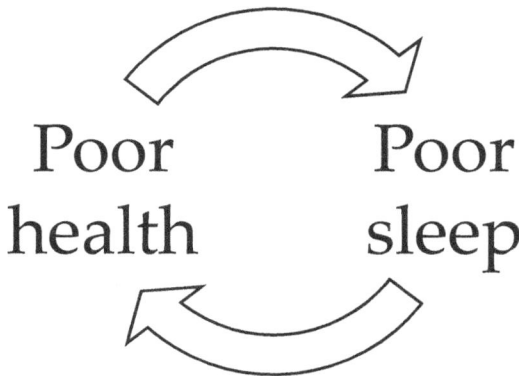

Poor
health
Poor
sleep

How to improve sleep

The effects of sleep on health, as well as the impact of various aspects of health on sleep, are clear. A substantial body of research suggests that this relationship is bidirectional, and there are numerous ways to improve both sleep and overall health.

Eat a healthy diet

Healthy diets that focus on a mostly unrefined selection of foods (like the Mediterranean Diet) promote longer and better-quality sleep,[138-140] and this is especially true when they include more fruits and vegetables. Conversely, diets higher in sugar, sweets, and snacks are associated with reduced sleep quality.[141] Ultra-refined foods, on the other hand, are associated with obesity, and this is known to also affect sleep.[141,142]

Meals are usually better than 'snacks'

Missing main meals and snacking are associated with worsened diet quality *and* poorer sleep.[141,143] So, instead, we should focus on eating good, healthy meals until we are full, and then eat again (a healthy, well-balanced meal) when we are hungry, rather than snacking.

Eat plenty of protein and veggies

Vegetables are associated with improved sleep,[144-146] as are adequate protein intakes.[144] You don't need to go overboard with this, as very high protein intakes don't necessarily improve sleep further.[147]

Eat 2-3+ fist-sized serves of vegetables at each meal and 1-2 palm-sized serves of a protein food.

Morning light

Human circadian rhythms are influenced heavily by light and dark cycles. When it is lighter, we wake up, and when it is darker, we tend towards sleep. This light exposure acts as a *zeitgeber*: a natural cue that initiates appropriate circadian rhythms.[148]

Meta-analysis has shown that exposure to bright light earlier in the day can improve sleep duration, reduce general sleep disturbances, and decrease insomnia and Alzheimer's-related sleep disturbances.[149]

Exposure to high lux levels (a measure of light intensity) of morning sunlight is crucial for regulating our circadian rhythm, which influences sleep patterns, mood, and alertness throughout the day. The intensity of natural light, particularly in the morning, signals to our bodies that it is time to wake up and be active. The much lower lux levels of indoor lighting are often insufficient to provide this strong biological cue.

Light Source	Typical Lux Levels
Direct morning sunlight	32,000 - 100,000+ lux
Ambient daylight (morning)	10,000 - 25,000 lux
Overcast day	1,000 - 2,000 lux
Well-lit office	300 - 500 lux
Home living room	100 - 300 lux

While any brighter-than-normal light exposure in the morning improves sleep,[150] natural sunlight (as shown in the table above) is much brighter and provides a far greater stimulus. Research also suggests that natural sunlight reduces the adverse effects of evening artificial light exposure on sleep.[151]

So, sitting in front of a computer screen or your phone under indoor lighting just doesn't cut it... Outdoor, full-spectrum sunlight is an underappreciated super-tactic to improve sleep.

Get outdoors, in natural light, for 5-15 minutes every morning.

Midday sun

Midday sun is also helpful for sleep quality. Vitamin D helps to regulate the sleep-wake cycle,[148,152] and getting out into the sun helps provide a one-two punch for improving sleep by providing the light-derived 'trigger' for proper regulation of our sleep-wake cycle, as well as the vitamin D-related effects on circadian rhythms.

If we can't get out in the sun all the time, or during winter when vitamin D production from sun exposure is lower, taking a vitamin D supplement can also help to preserve vitamin D levels and improve sleep duration and quality.[153,154] One key caveat is that **you should never burn.** Adjust your sun exposure accordingly and be sun smart!

Get out in the sun with your face, torso, arms, and legs (or more!) exposed for 10 minutes per day, and/or take a vitamin D supplement (~2000 IU per day).

Note: Vitamin D dosing varies considerably. For specific dosing advice, consult a qualified and registered nutritionist or dietitian.

Consider zinc and magnesium before bed

Magnesium helps reduce excessive nerve firing and is considered our primary 'relaxing' mineral[155] which can improve sleep.[156] Magnesium is likely to both improve sleep and reduce drowsiness, while low magnesium levels worsen sleep.[157-160] It can also mitigate some of the adverse effects on performance from insufficient sleep.[161] Magnesium supplementation specifically has been shown to benefit sleep.[162]

Similarly, zinc is involved in many hundreds of enzymatic reactions in the body, some of which are critical to sleep cycles. Zinc supplementation and higher intakes of zinc-rich foods can improve both the quantity and quality of sleep.[163-165]

If you're having trouble sleeping, consider a zinc/magnesium supplement containing ~400 mg magnesium and 15 mg zinc.

Consult a qualified and registered nutrition practitioner before considering supplementing with specific nutrients.

Note: A great way to get sufficient zinc and magnesium is within a quality multi-vitamin that also includes ~900 mcg of copper (which is vital to have 'in balance' with zinc)

Meditate before bed

Mindfulness and meditation target key risk factors of poor sleep, such as awareness, control, and, most importantly, acceptance (especially of the things you can't control).[166]

Meditative practices, such as 'mindfulness-based stress reduction' (a meditation practice originally derived from Buddhist practice and now used as a medical intervention), are likely to improve sleep quality as much as, or even more than, other active interventions, and more than passive 'control' actions.[167–169]

Similarly, mindful movement practices such as meditation, yoga, chi gong, and Pilates have been shown to have beneficial effects on sleep quality, along with improvements in quality of life, physical performance, and depression,[170,171] and they might help to reduce chronic pain and improve sleep quality in people with chronic illness.[172]

Use mindfulness of breath meditation before bed (or take up another mindfulness practice like yoga or qi gong)

Get more (and earlier) sleep

A clear link exists between reduced sleep duration and poorer health. For example, while napping can help to reduce sleep debt, longer sleep is preferable for improving performance. [173] Interestingly, while we often hear advice that 'banking' sleep is ineffective (i.e., getting more sleep before or after a period of reduced sleep), a systematic review of sleep patterns among shift workers has suggested that banking sleep before shift work can help improve safety, performance, and reduce fatigue.[174]

Try going to bed ½ an hour or more earlier than usual and notice any differences in your waking and daily energy and mental performance.

Have a warm bath or shower before bed

Taking a warm bath or shower increases body temperature, resulting in greater peripheral blood flow and vasodilation to help return it to normal levels. The subsequent temperature drop after taking a bath or shower is thought to help induce sleep and increase the release of sleep-inducing hormones, such as melatonin. This is because it mimics one of the 'sleep signals' of our circadian rhythm – the inevitable cooling of the environment as the sun sets.

A bath or shower at 40-42.5 degrees Celsius has been shown to improve sleep quality and reduce the time it takes to fall asleep when taken approximately 1-2 hours before bed.[175]

If you're having trouble sleeping, try having a warm bath or shower before bed.

Exercise

Exercise improves sleep quality, duration, and the time it takes to fall asleep.[176-179] In particular, exercise is an effective way to help combat insomnia.[179,180] Exercising in the evening also helps, rather than hinders, overall sleep duration and quality. However, vigorous exercise less than an hour before bed can reduce sleep duration, increase the time it takes to fall asleep, and negatively impact sleep quality.[181] In a 2017 review of intervention studies, 29 of 34 studies concluded that exercise improved either sleep duration or quality,[177] and in a meta-analysis from the same year, a significant improvement in sleep was seen with exercise.[176]

Resistance exercise

Most of the recent reviews have focused on aerobic or mindful exercise regimens. A recent review of the effects of resistance training (weight training) found that consistent resistance exercise improves all aspects of sleep, with the greatest benefit being observed in sleep quality. The review also suggests that resistance exercise may improve anxiety and depression.[182]

Establish a habit of regular exercise, including strength training, but be mindful of exercising intensely too close to bedtime.

Reduce use of screen devices and exposure to media...

There is a strong and consistent association between the bedtime use of screen devices, such as phones and tablets, and inadequate sleep, poor sleep quality, and excessive daytime sleepiness.[183] There is a greater than two-fold increased risk of having sleep problems if you compulsively use the internet ('internet addiction').[184]

Turn off your phone at least two hours before bedtime and limit your exposure to excessive nighttime light.

Reduce caffeine

Caffeinated beverages have health benefits and can help improve cognition and reduce the risk of neurodegenerative disorders,[112,113,185] but excessive use or use late in the day can reduce sleep quality and duration. Additionally, slow-wave sleep, which is crucial for the body's recovery and repair, is diminished, while sleep arousal is increased.

Several factors influence the effect of caffeine on sleep, with the timing of intake and dosage being the most important. Additionally, older adults may be more sensitive to these effects than younger people. There is also significant genetic variation in tolerance to caffeine.[186]

Restrict caffeine to the morning, and if you're having trouble sleeping, reduce your intake of coffee, tea, and/or cocoa.

Limit alcohol

Higher intakes of alcohol consumption increase the risk of sleep apnoea and reduce the quality of sleep.[187]

Stick to the best health guidelines for alcohol (less than 3-5 drinks per week) and avoid drinking more than three drinks on any given day.

Reduce noise

Noise (such as road or aircraft noise) can affect sleep quality.[188]

Look into deeper reasons for sleep disturbances

Inflicted trauma, including sexual violence and abuse, physical violence, or psychological aggression, is known to increase sleep disturbance.[189] Interventions (some of which have been mentioned above), such as improved 'sleep hygiene', cognitive behavioural therapy, mindfulness and relaxation practices, and psychotherapy and hypnotherapy, can help us to deal with trauma and improve sleep.[190] Cognitive behavioural therapy shows particularly strong effects for improving sleep,[190] although these effects seem to be primarily related to subjective (self-reported) rather than laboratory measures of sleep.[191]

Sleep: A summary

Sleep has a significant and bidirectional effect on health, meaning that the worse you sleep, the worse your health and vice versa. To enhance health and performance, prioritising sleep should be a goal. To improve sleep, we need to establish 'sleep rituals.' These sleep rituals, often referred to as 'sleep hygiene practices,' have been shown to enhance sleep quality and duration.[190]

Sleep tactics

- Get outside for 5-15 minutes to experience full-spectrum light exposure
- Get to bed at a time that allows at least 7 hours of total sleep before waking
    o This time should be extended if you are being woken by an alarm every morning or if you are waking exhausted
- Reduce alcohol intake to safe levels (i.e. <3-5 drinks per week) and eliminate caffeine in the afternoon
- Avoid screen use for 1-2 hours before going to bed
- Limit social media use in the evening
- Exercise according to your recovery ability
- Use meditation, mindfulness, a hot shower, or a cup of relaxing herbal tea to help induce sleep
- If past trauma is a reason for poor sleep, consider seeing a counsellor, psychotherapist, psychiatrist, or psychologist experienced in trauma counselling

13

STRESS

Stress and its responses are a natural part of our ability to survive and thrive. However, both acute and chronic stress that cannot be reconciled and recovered from result in lasting health implications and excessive stress is related to poor health, pain, loss of quality of life, increased risk of cancer and cardiovascular disease, and worsened all-cause mortality. Thousands of papers have been written on the effects of stress on health. The undeniable impact of stress on many health outcomes is often overlooked in many areas of clinical practice, receiving only token appreciation.

What is stress?

In this context, we mean stress in the *psychoneurophysiological* (mind-body) context. In other words, the stressors that we usually think of as psychological exert effects on the body (and vice versa). Stress is the body's response to any stimulus or challenge. The stressor is typically a threat, and so, the body responds to the presence of a threat (or challenge) with chemical and structural changes to allow us to respond appropriately.

The two major systems that respond to stress are the autonomic nervous system and the hypothalamic-pituitary-adrenal (HPA) axis.

The sympathoadrenal medullary (SAM) axis activates the fight-or-flight response through the sympathetic nervous system, which dedicates energy to relevant body systems (such as the working muscles to enable you to run away from a tiger). Once the threat is effectively dealt with, the parasympathetic nervous system ('rest and digest') returns the body to homeostasis. Secondarily, the HPA axis regulates the release of cortisol, which exerts influence on metabolic, psychological, and immune functions. These various mechanisms, when combined, allow the actions to resolve the threat while also interplaying with our innate reward system, memory and cognition, immune function, and metabolic state. Nowadays, most of the stressors we encounter are not life-threatening (although they may be socially significant), but our responses remain the same.

Life stress has a range of physical effects and, similarly to any other stressor, influences the HPA axis, hypothalamic-pituitary-gonadal axis, SAM axis, and the immune system.[192] Severe or repeated life-stressors that cannot be adequately reconciled mentally, and that we can't recover from physically, can result in severe stress-related effects, including 'burnout' and chronic fatigue,[193] and even worrying *about* stressful events increases the amount of 'wear and tear' on the mind and body.[194]

Chronic stress is involved in the development and severity of many mental and physical conditions, including asthma, rheumatoid arthritis, anxiety disorders, depression, cardiovascular disease, chronic pain, human immunodeficiency virus/AIDS, stroke, and cancer.[195]

Acute stressors (like work-related incidents in hospitals) can induce long-term post-traumatic stress disorder (PTSD), depression, and anxiety,[196] and severe traumas (such as abuse when young) can also result in an increase in health problems overall and an increase in pain associated with health conditions.[197]

Acute stressors and trauma can result in[198]:

- poor general physical health
- increased pain and disability
- lower quality of life
- higher risk of all-cause mortality
- increased rates of depression and anxiety
- psychosocial outcomes (e.g. increased family conflict)

Stress responses that are not properly modulated (resulting in either excessive or insufficient stress reactions to stimuli) negatively affect health later in life.[199]

The role of work-related stress in health

Work stress is associated with a 50% increase in the risk of cardiovascular disease.[200] The amount of work and even the amount of stress are not the most important factors, though. The 'effort-to-reward' imbalance is the biggest predictor of adverse effects from stress. In other words, if the perceived reward from work is not proportionate to the effort of work, the stress effect is amplified.

Similarly, overcommitment to tasks is also related to increased stress and poorer cardiovascular health outcomes. Poorer reward-to-effort ratios are also associated with high blood pressure and arterial thickening.[200]

Stress & body composition

Reviews of the evidence indicate a strong bidirectional relationship between stress, sleep, and food intake. In other words, stress worsens sleep and increases food intake, resulting in weight gain. Additionally, worsened sleep drives poorer food choices, which in turn worsen sleep, creating a vicious cycle. Obesity is a known risk factor for sleep disorders.[76]

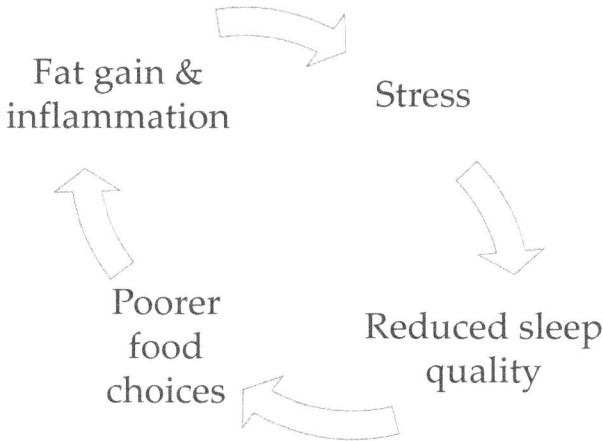

Fat gain & inflammation

Stress

Poorer food choices

Reduced sleep quality

Chronic stress promotes a shift to overeating. This contrasts with acute stress, which often reduces food intake (because appetite-suppressing stress hormones). Hyperactivation of stress responses promotes metabolic shifts that encourage fat gain and increase inflammation, which in turn is associated with further fat gain. Detrimental changes also occur in the gut microbiota, which may contribute to a trend toward adiposity.[77]

Research has demonstrated that in working-age adults, high job demands and work stress are associated with up to 30% greater weight gain,[201-203] and men who are already overweight might be more at risk of stress-driven fat gain.[78]

How to deal with stress

As we have already discussed, one of the most significant stress factors is the work-reward ratio of your job. So, having a better relationship with not just your work, but your life and where it is heading, is critical to reducing stress. We all know what it's like to feel directionless and without a sense of purpose. That's why finding your **why** and aligning your life with your **ethos** is so important (as we covered earlier in the book).

Additionally, simply taking care of the foundations of health (through diet, exercise, and sleep) helps you to become far more resilient in the face of life's stressors.

Finally, directly stress-reducing methods, such as taking time off, engaging in hobbies, and participating in relaxing activities like yoga or tai chi, all help to mitigate the effects of stress.

Of particular value is meditation, as we have introduced in the chapter on Sleep. Interestingly, evidence suggests that even brief meditations (around 10 minutes per day) are equally effective in reducing psychological distress and improving well-being when compared to longer sessions of 30 minutes or more per day.[204,205] Most of the beneficial effects of meditation are seen *on the day of meditation,*[206] and beneficial results increase over time.[207]

Therefore, consistency of practice, even if you are doing short meditations of 10 minutes per day, is far more effective than trying to do long sessions but failing to do so consistently. I highly suggest sticking to 10 minutes every day until you establish a strong habit of meditation. Then, consider increasing the duration, but only if you wish.

How to meditate

The 'One Minute Meditation Challenge'

When I ask clients if they meditate, the most common answer I get is "No... But I know I *should*."

Firstly, 'should' is bullshit. Either do or don't, there ain't no 'should' around here...

People recognise that meditation is valuable, but they struggle to apply it and create the habit of *doing it* every day. Many people don't feel that they have enough time, yet they often find themselves procrastinating, watching YouTube videos, and doomscrolling for far longer than it would take to just meditate!

Therefore, we need to create a habit, and the most effective way to do this is to start small and practice it every day.

I typically ask my clients if they have just one minute to devote to meditation the next day.

One minute? *One minute?!* They say...

Yes, just one minute!

When we start with one minute and build minute-by-minute over consecutive days, we are training our 'meditation muscle' just as

208

we'd train for physical strength by increasing the repetitions and load that we use over time.

Start with one minute of mindfulness of breath tomorrow, then increase your meditation by one minute each day until you are doing ten minutes. Aim for at least 30 unbroken days of meditation.

Mindfulness of breath

- Find a quiet, comfortable place to sit.
- Sit with your back straight and upright, not rigidly but with good posture. You may like to use a traditional posture, such as a lotus or half-lotus position, or sit on your heels with your knees folded under you. These postures were developed for meditation and are highly effective in promoting relaxation and mental clarity. You can also sit in a comfortable chair with your heels flat on the floor and your back supported, keeping it upright.
- Place your hands together comfortably in your lap.
- Close your eyes – but not tightly.
- Begin breathing in and out through your nose. Do not 'try' to breathe deeply or in any fashion; breathe comfortably and without effort.
- Notice the sensation of the air passing in and out of your nose. There will be a point or area in your nostrils or on the outside rim where you will feel the breath as it moves in and out. Gently bring your attention to this area.

Note: You may find it helpful to count your breaths initially. Count each in and out breath as one breath, and count your breaths up to 10 if you find that this enables you to get into the meditation.

- Keep 'watching' the breath; when your mind wanders, bring it back gently to the point where you can feel the breath. It's that simple...

I have used the *Mindfulness* app and Insight Timer to time my meditations (available on Apple and Android).

Meditation summary

- Start with a one-minute meditation first thing tomorrow morning.
- Add one minute each day until you reach 10 minutes.
- Meditate each day for 6 weeks straight.
- Don't break the chain!

14

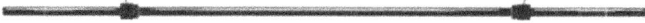

THE AA40 DAY

Putting it all together

As health and performance practitioners, Daz and I often get asked what we do and what our days consist of. While blindly following someone else's schedule is seldom a good idea (because each of us has a distinct set of life circumstances), one can gain insight into structuring one's own day by examining the tactics others use to achieve health and life success.

So, take the following with a pinch of salt... These are not THE way to structure your day; they are simply the ways that Daz and I structure ours.

Cliff's day

Time	Activity	Food/Drink/Supplement/Notes
6 am	Get up with the kids	Water A shake with Nuzest Good Green Vitality, egg white protein & collagen (~30 g protein), N-acetyl cysteine. Sometimes extra magnesium, added vitamin D (2000 IU+) in winter, and Coffee.
8 am	Training	6-10 min mobility, 30-40 min strength training) or Jiu Jitsu 2-3 days of the week
9 am	After training	Post Workout drink with 1 scoop of whey protein, 400 ml high-protein milk, and 1 tsp creatine
12 pm	Lunch	~150 g meat, veggies, carbs (amount varies depending on goals). I also have some vitamin C with lunch.
3 pm	Shake	Same as post-workout
6 pm	Dinner with family	Like lunch, usually more veggies and carbohydrates, and 'freer' carbs (like Ramen)
After dinner		High protein milk, dates, berries, yoghurt, a small amount of white chocolate, cookies, or another 'treat'

Daz's day

Over the years, the things I have tried to make non-negotiable parts of my day have ebbed and flowed, but a few key elements have always remained constant, anchoring me.

1. Joint circles

From gymnastics as a 5-year-old to martial arts in my teens, we began our training sessions by incorporating movement through the joints, increasing the flow of synovial fluid, exploring the range of motion, and checking for restrictions or pain. While it's not a guaranteed daily practice, it has been the most consistent over the years - 5 minutes is all it takes, from neck to ankles; my body immediately feels 10 times better, and I'm ready to take on the day. If I have more time, I'll build on it with a movement flow that takes the joints through more challenging positions with the added benefits of coordination, core stability, and balance work.

I try to make it the first thing I do out of bed, and it's (almost) as good as coffee....

2. Coffee

Say no more.

Ok, just a little more. The stimulant benefit aside, I enjoy the ritual of it. I'm typically the first in the household to wake, and those few quiet moments are a great chance for reflection on the previous day, a little gratitude, and some planning for the day ahead.

3. Dawn walk

I never really was one for walking, but at the same time, it's one of the most potent things we can do for our health.

So, I walk.

It helps if you can find a trail or a beach, or an interesting neighbourhood to walk through. Pandemic lockdowns, along with having a dog and a new baby, have helped me double my average daily steps, and I hope to maintain this habit long-term.

The morning sun on your face boosts your mood with a strong shot of serotonin, increases Vitamin D, which plays a role in immune health, and helps stabilise your circadian rhythm for better sleep quality at the end of the day.

4. Play

I've always looked younger than my years (although it has evened out recently). I've also acted younger. Whether that was delaying adult responsibility in my 20s as I "wandered the earth like Caine from Kung Fu, meeting people and having adventures" or simply not being afraid to act the fool. This is a significant issue for adults, particularly in my native New Zealand, where I often see people choosing to avoid trying something new so they won't look silly.

Forget that!

Balance-beam-walk on the curb, climb a tree, do handstands and cartwheels and bear crawls in the park, chase your kids or your dog,

Do we stop playing because we get old, or do we get old because we stop playing?

5. Movement

Now, it's essential to note that by ticking the above boxes, I have already made some progress. And by front-loading the above, it helps to guarantee a minimum effective dose just in case the rest of the day turns to custard, and I can avoid beating myself up about missing a workout. But if things are going well, I try to alternate between days of either a formalised strength training workout or a more aerobic-style session outdoors, such as mountain biking, ocean swimming, surfing, or paddleboarding. I'm forever trying to make Jiu Jitsu a regular part of my week too, but I'm not there yet...

15

AWESOME AFTER IN 40 WORDS

Eat real food.

Prioritise sleep.

Manage stress.

Walk daily.

Lift weights, practice gymnastics, bike, swim, run.

Emphasise range of motion and technique above load and volume.

Learn new activities, outdoors preferably.

Train with friends.

Get a coach.

Make it fun.

THE AUTHORS

Darren Ellis MSc

Darren "Daz" Ellis didn't set out to be a fitness coach. After flunking high school, he worked in restaurants, farms, and nightclub doors to fund adventures through Africa, Asia, and the Middle East.

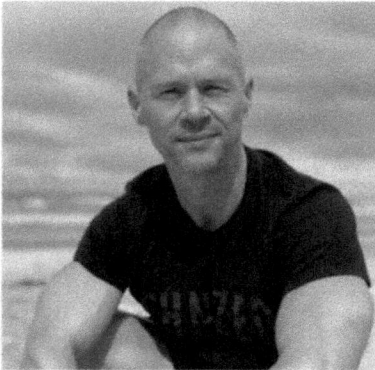

But at 25, the quarter-life crisis hit, and he returned to NZ to study, eventually earning a master's degree in Exercise Physiology.

Realising quickly that there was no "Exercise Physiologists Wanted" column in the situations vacant, he built his own path. From gym shifts to outdoor boot camps and then opening New Zealand's first CrossFit affiliate (back when people thought "CrossFit" was just being angry about exercise...). He even competed at the CrossFit Games both as a team member and as a master's athlete.

But over the years (and especially once becoming a father), Daz saw a truth most of the fitness industry ignores: lifelong fitness is different from world-class fitness. Busy, over-40 adults don't need gruelling, soul-crushing workouts. They need a practice that complements their life rather than consumes it.

Today, with over two decades of coaching and thousands of clients, Daz is recognised for his minimalist fitness approach, with methods designed for real life rather than elite performance. His programs help regular people build muscle, move well, and stay resilient with time-efficient, sustainable training that fits around work, family, and the things they love.

Part coach, part industry bullcrap translator, Daz aims to blend proven science with practical application. His belief is simple: the best workouts should make you feel better, not worse, and they should be something you can keep doing forever, not just for a holiday six-pack.

In this book, he shares the lessons, strategies, and mindset shifts to help you stay strong, mobile, and adventurous, well beyond your 40s. Find him at **www.darrenellis.coach**

Cliff Harvey PhD

Dr Cliff Harvey is a nutritionist, strength and conditioning coach, and former World Champion lifter. But if you want to know who he really is, you should know about the nail-polish and skirt-wearing captain of his high school's 1st XV rugby team.

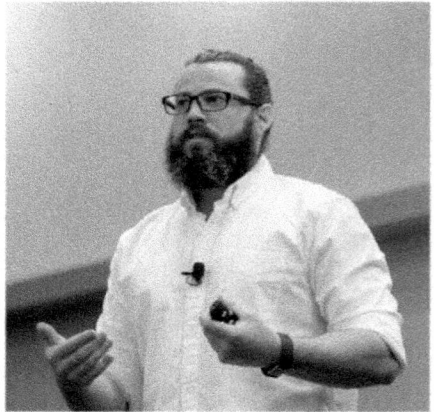

Cliff has always been a walking contradiction. He's the researcher who knows he knows "jack-shit," the jock who rebelled, and the seeker who found his passion for the human body mostly to prove to his Mum that he could amount to something.

That mission became the driving force of his life, but she never got to see it fulfilled. The night before he opened his first business, his Mum passed away from an asthma attack as he tried, unsuccessfully, to revive her.

That single event sent him spiralling. He built a hugely successful business by day and burned it all down by night, fuelled by grief, anger, and anything else that could dull the pain. He was the right guy at the right time doing all the right things in business—and all the wrong things in life. The inevitable crash came in the form of chronic fatigue so severe that he could barely get out of bed. It was a forced re-evaluation that cost him his business and his health, but it gave him his first real lesson in what *truly* sustainable practice looks like.

His own body has been his most challenging research project. Juggling a bipolar 2 diagnosis, Crohn's disease, and autoimmune issues, he's had to be more than a textbook academic. He became a practitioner of resilience, testing his methods in the real world not only to manage his health but also to win world titles and records in All-Round Weightlifting. He helped thousands of others achieve their goals, ranging from winning Olympic medals to overcoming the effects of chronic illness.

At his core, Cliff believes that the ultimate goal is to live a healthier, happier life while helping others do the same. He's not a guru who thinks enlightenment is just around the corner; he's a seeker who has been punched in the face, held up at gunpoint, won, lost, and carried his mother's coffin. He knows the weight of real life.

In this book, he shares the hard-won lessons from that life, blending science with the simple, powerful truth that your health should complement your world, not consume it.

www.holisticperformance.institute

www.cliffharvey.com

REFERENCES

1. Aune D, Sen A, ó'Hartaigh B, Janszky I, Romundstad PR, Tonstad S, et al. Resting heart rate and the risk of cardiovascular disease, total cancer, and all-cause mortality – A systematic review and dose–response meta-analysis of prospective studies. Nutrition, Metabolism and Cardiovascular Diseases [Internet]. 2017 June 1;27(6):504–17. Available from: https://www.sciencedirect.com/science/article/pii/S0939475317 300856

2. Ashwell M, Gunn P, Gibson S. Waist-to-height ratio is a better screening tool than waist circumference and BMI for adult cardiometabolic risk factors: systematic review and meta-analysis. Obesity Reviews [Internet]. 2012 Mar 1;13(3):275–86. Available from: https://doi.org/10.1111/j.1467-789X.2011.00952.x

3. Ashwell M, Mayhew L, Richardson J, Rickayzen B. Waist-to-height ratio is more predictive of years of life lost than body mass index. PLoS One [Internet]. 2011 Sept 8;9(9):e103483. Available from: http://www.ncbi.nlm.nih.gov/pmc/articles/PMC4157748/

4. Browning LM, Hsieh SD, Ashwell M. A systematic review of waist-to-height ratio as a screening tool for the prediction of cardiovascular disease and diabetes: 0·5 could be a suitable global boundary value. Nutrition Research Reviews [Internet]. 2010;23(2):247–69. Available from:

https://www.cambridge.org/core/article/systematic-review-of-waisttoheight-ratio-as-a-screening-tool-for-the-prediction-of-cardiovascular-disease-and-diabetes-05-could-be-a-suitable-global-boundary-value/A65EC8CCE2A120C247F82C5074C24C7D

5. Corrêa MM, Thumé E, De Oliveira ERA, Tomasi E. Performance of the waist-to-height ratio in identifying obesity and predicting non-communicable diseases in the elderly population: A systematic literature review. Archives of Gerontology and Geriatrics [Internet]. 2016 July 1;65:174–82. Available from: https://www.sciencedirect.com/science/article/pii/S0167494316 300619

6. Mazur LJ, Yetman RJ, Risser WL. Weight-training injuries. Common injuries and preventative methods. Sports Med [Internet]. 1993;16(1):57–63. Available from: http://dx.doi.org/10.2165/00007256-199316010-00005

7. Carroll KM, Bazyler CD, Bernards JR, Taber CB, Stuart CA, DeWeese BH, et al. Skeletal Muscle Fiber Adaptations Following Resistance Training Using Repetition Maximums or Relative Intensity. Sports (Basel) [Internet]. 2019;7(7). Available from: http://dx.doi.org/10.3390/sports7070169

8. Santanielo N, Nóbrega SR, Scarpelli MC, Alvarez IF, Otoboni GB, Pintanel L, et al. Effect of resistance training to muscle failure vs non-failure on strength, hypertrophy and muscle architecture in trained individuals. Biol Sport [Internet]. 2020;37(4):333–41. Available from: http://dx.doi.org/10.5114/biolsport.2020.96317

9. Andersen V, Paulsen G, Stien N, Baarholm M, Seynnes O, Saeterbakken AH. Resistance Training With Different Velocity Loss Thresholds Induce Similar Changes in Strengh and Hypertrophy. J Strength Cond Res [Internet]. 2021; Available from: http://dx.doi.org/10.1519/jsc.0000000000004067

10. Iversen VM, Norum M, Schoenfeld BJ, Fimland MS. No Time to Lift? Designing Time-Efficient Training Programs for Strength and Hypertrophy: A Narrative Review. Sports Medicine [Internet]. 2021 Oct 1;51(10):2079–95. Available from: https://doi.org/10.1007/s40279-021-01490-1

11. Krzysztofik M, Wilk M, Wojdała G, Gołaś A. Maximizing Muscle Hypertrophy: A Systematic Review of Advanced Resistance Training Techniques and Methods. International journal of environmental research and public health [Internet]. 2019;16(24):4897. Available from: https://www.ncbi.nlm.nih.gov/pmc/articles/PMC6950543/

12. Pelland J, Remmert J, Robinson Z, Hinson S, Zourdos M. The resistance training dose-response: Meta-regressions exploring the effects of weekly volume and frequency on muscle hypertrophy and strength gain [Internet]. 2024 [cited 2024 Oct 9]. Available from: https://sportrxiv.org/index.php/server/preprint/view/460

13. McMaster DT, Gill N, Cronin J, McGuigan M. The development, retention and decay rates of strength and power in elite rugby union, rugby league and American football: a systematic review. Sports Med [Internet]. 2013;43(5):367–84. Available from: http://dx.doi.org/10.1007/s40279-013-0031-3

14. Afonso J, Ramirez-Campillo R, Moscão J, Rocha T, Zacca R, Martins A, et al. Strength Training versus Stretching for Improving Range of Motion: A Systematic Review and Meta-Analysis. Healthcare (Basel, Switzerland) [Internet]. 2021;9(4):427. Available from: https://www.ncbi.nlm.nih.gov/pmc/articles/PMC8067745/

15. Shamus E, Shamus J. Sports injury: prevention & rehabilitation. McGraw-Hill New York; 2001.

16. Leech J, Andrew K. The emerging prominence of nutrition in injury management. Sport Health. 2013;31(1):57.

17. Medina D, Lizarraga A, Drobnick F. Injury prevention and nutrition in football. Sports Sci Exchange. 2014;27(132):1–5.

18. Kloubec J, Harris C. WHOLE FOODS NUTRITION FOR ENHANCED INJURY PREVENTION AND HEALING. ACSM's Health & Fitness Journal [Internet]. 2016;20(2):7–11. Available from: https://journals.lww.com/acsm-healthfitness/Fulltext/2016/03000/WHOLE_FOODS_NUTRITION_FOR_ENHANCED_INJURY.5.aspx

19. Caldwell SB, Smith D, Wilson FC. Impact of paroxysmal sympathetic hyperactivity on nutrition management after brain injury: A case series. Brain Injury [Internet]. 2014 Mar 1;28(3):370–3. Available from: https://doi.org/10.3109/02699052.2013.865265

20. Härtl R, Gerber LM, Ni Q, Ghajar J. Effect of early nutrition on deaths due to severe traumatic brain injury. Journal of neurosurgery. 2008;109(1):50–6.

21. White H, Venkatesh B. Clinical review: ketones and brain injury. Critical Care [Internet]. 2011;15(2):219–219. Available from: http://www.ncbi.nlm.nih.gov/pmc/articles/PMC3219306/

22. Guzmán M, Blázquez C. Ketone body synthesis in the brain: possible neuroprotective effects. Prostaglandins, Leukotrienes and Essential Fatty Acids [Internet]. 2004 Mar 1;70(3):287–92. Available from: http://www.sciencedirect.com/science/article/pii/S0952327803002199

23. Xu K, LaManna JC, Puchowicz MA. Neuroprotective Properties of Ketone Bodies. Wolf M, Bucher HU, Rudin M, Van Huffel S, Wolf U, Bruley DF, et al., editors. Springer New York; 2012. 97–102 p.

24. Tai KK, Nguyen N, Pham L, Truong DD. Ketogenic diet prevents cardiac arrest-induced cerebral ischemic neurodegeneration. Journal of Neural Transmission [Internet]. 2008 July 1;115(7):1011–7. Available from: https://doi.org/10.1007/s00702-008-0050-7

25. Schutz PW. Neuroprotective effects of ketone bodies during hypoglycemia. University of British Columbia; 2011.

26. Hertz L, Chen Y, Waagepetersen HS. Effects of ketone bodies in Alzheimer's disease in relation to neural hypometabolism, β-amyloid toxicity, and astrocyte function. Journal Of Neurochemistry [Internet]. 2015;134(1):7–20. Available from: http://search.ebscohost.com/login.aspx?direct=true&db=mdc&AN=25832906&site=ehost-live

27. Youm YH, Nguyen KY, Grant RW, Goldberg EL, Bodogai M, Kim D, et al. The ketone metabolite β-hydroxybutyrate blocks NLRP3 inflammasome-mediated inflammatory disease. Nat Med [Internet]. 2015;21(3):263–9. Available from: http://search.ebscohost.com/login.aspx?direct=true&db=mdc&AN=25686106&site=ehost-live

28. Gzielo K, Soltys Z, Rajfur Z, Setkowicz ZK. The Impact of the Ketogenic Diet on Glial Cells Morphology. A Quantitative Morphological Analysis. Neuroscience [Internet]. 2019 June 18; Available from: http://www.sciencedirect.com/science/article/pii/S0306452219304154

29. Choragiewicz TJ, Thaler S, Rejdak R, Fiedorowoicz M, Turski WA, Kocki T, et al. Neuroprotective Effect of Ketone Bodies and Ketogenic Diet in Nmda-Induced Rgc Damage in Rat. Possible Involvement of Kynurenic Acid? Investigative Ophthalmology & Visual Science [Internet]. 2010;51(13):3715–3715. Available from: http://dx.doi.org/

30. Kim SW, Marosi K, Mattson M. Ketone beta-hydroxybutyrate up-regulates BDNF expression through NF-κB as an adaptive response against ROS, which may improve neuronal bioenergetics and enhance neuroprotection (P3.090). Neurology. 2017;88(16 Supplement).

31. Lai PL, Naidu M, Sabaratnam V, Wong KH, David RP, Kuppusamy UR, et al. Neurotrophic Properties of the Lion's Mane Medicinal Mushroom, *Hericium erinaceus* (Higher Basidiomycetes) from Malaysia. 2013 Nov 15;15(6):539–54. Available from: http://dl.begellhouse.com/journals/708ae68d64b17c52,034eeb 045436a171,750a15ad12ae25e9.html

32. Park YS, Lee HS, Won MH, Lee JH, Lee SY, Lee HY. Effect of an exo-polysaccharide from the culture broth of Hericium erinaceus on enhancement of growth and differentiation of rat adrenal nerve cells. Cytotechnology [Internet]. 2002 Sept 1;39(3):155. Available from: http://dx.doi.org/10.1023/A:1023963509393

33. Nagano M, Shimizu K, Kondo R, Hayashi C, Sato D, Kitagawa K, et al. Reduction of depression and anxiety by 4 weeks Hericium erinaceus intake. Biomedical Research [Internet]. 2010;31(4):231–7. Available from: http://dx.doi.org/10.2220/biomedres.31.231

34. Wong KH, Vikineswary S, Naidu M, Keynes R. Activity of Aqueous Extracts of Lion's Mane Mushroom *Hericium erinaceus* (Bull.: Fr.)

Pers. (Aphyllophoromycetideae) on the Neural Cell Line NG108-15. 2007 Mar 23;9(1):57–65. Available from: http://dl.begellhouse.com/journals/708ae68d64b17c52,0d49dda96a2a7147,6ce1a4f7295df1fb.html

35. Wong KH, Naidu M, David P, Abdulla MA, Abdullah N, Kuppusamy UR, et al. Peripheral Nerve Regeneration Following Crush Injury to Rat Peroneal Nerve by Aqueous Extract of Medicinal Mushroom Hericium erinaceus (Bull.: Fr) Pers. (Aphyllophoromycetideae). Evidence-Based Complementary and Alternative Medicine [Internet]. 2011;2011:10. Available from: http://dx.doi.org/10.1093/ecam/neq062

36. Wong KH, Naidu M, David RP, Abdulla MA, Kuppusamy UR. Functional Recovery Enhancement Following Injury to Rodent Peroneal Nerve by Lion's Mane Mushroom, *Hericium erinaceus* (Bull.: Fr.) Pers. (Aphyllophoromycetideae). 2009 Oct 1;11(3):225–36. Available from: http://dl.begellhouse.com/journals/708ae68d64b17c52,4f53a14232dd0d51,2faf43d457970ed7.html

37. Moldavan M, Grygansky AP, Kolotushkina OV, Kirchhoff B, Skibo GG, Pedarzani P. Neurotropic and Trophic Action of Lion's Mane Mushroom *Hericium erinaceus* (Bull.: Fr.) Pers. (Aphyllophoromycetideae) Extracts on Nerve Cells *in Vitro*. 2007 Mar 23;9(1):15–28. Available from: http://dl.begellhouse.com/journals/708ae68d64b17c52,0d49dda96a2a7147,504922782f5fa5ea.html

38. Mori K, Obara Y, Hirota M, Azumi Y, Kinugasa S, Inatomi S, et al. Nerve Growth Factor-Inducing Activity of *Hericium erinaceus* in 1321N1 Human Astrocytoma Cells. Biological and Pharmaceutical Bulletin [Internet]. 2008;31(9):1727–32. Available from: http://dx.doi.org/10.1248/bpb.31.1727

39. Peoples GE, McLennan PL. Fish oil for physical performance in athletes. In: Fish and Fish Oil in Health and Disease Prevention. Elsevier; 2016. p. 119–36.

40. Marques CG, Santos VC, Levada-Pires AC, Jacintho TM, Gorjão R, Pithon-Curi TC, et al. Effects of DHA-rich fish oil supplementation on the lipid profile, markers of muscle damage, and neutrophil function in wheelchair basketball athletes before and after acute exercise. Applied Physiology, Nutrition, and Metabolism. 2015;40(6):596–604.

41. Shin SS, Dixon CE. Oral fish oil restores striatal dopamine release after traumatic brain injury. Neuroscience Letters [Internet]. 2011 June 8;496(3):168–71. Available from: http://www.sciencedirect.com/science/article/pii/S0304394011004435

42. Zhang YM, Liu JC, Wang JB, Huang ZS, Tang H, Sun WJ. Effects of fish oil fatty acids on systemic inflammatory response syndrome after traumatic brain injury [J]. Parenteral & Enteral Nutrition. 2010;6.

43. Xu JG, Pan YJ, Zhao J. Effect of ω-3 fish oil fatty emulsion in patients with severe injury. Strait Pharmaceutical Journal. 2008;(8):51.

44. Song H, Li B. Beneficial effects of collagen hydrolysate: a review on recent developments. Biomed J Sci Technol Res. 2017;1–4.

45. Moskowitz RW. Role of collagen hydrolysate in bone and joint disease. Seminars in Arthritis and Rheumatism [Internet]. 2000 Oct 1;30(2):87–99. Available from: http://www.sciencedirect.com/science/article/pii/S004901720056 8255

46. Shigemura Y, Kubomura D, Sato Y, Sato K. Dose-dependent changes in the levels of free and peptide forms of hydroxyproline in human plasma after collagen hydrolysate ingestion. Food Chemistry [Internet]. 2014 Sept 15;159:328–32. Available from: http://www.sciencedirect.com/science/article/pii/S0308814614002763

47. Sugihara F, Inoue N, Kuwamori M, Taniguchi M. Quantification of hydroxyprolyl-glycine (Hyp-Gly) in human blood after ingestion of collagen hydrolysate. Journal of Bioscience and Bioengineering [Internet]. 2012 Feb 1;113(2):202–3. Available from: http://www.sciencedirect.com/science/article/pii/S1389172311003975

48. Bello AE, Oesser S. Collagen hydrolysate for the treatment of osteoarthritis and other joint disorders:a review of the literature. Current Medical Research and Opinion [Internet]. 2006 Nov 1;22(11):2221–32. Available from: https://doi.org/10.1185/030079906X148373

49. Bruyère O, Zegels B, Leonori L, Rabenda V, Janssen A, Bourges C, et al. Effect of collagen hydrolysate in articular pain: A 6-month randomized, double-blind, placebo controlled study. Complementary Therapies in Medicine [Internet]. 2012 June 1;20(3):124–30. Available from: http://www.sciencedirect.com/science/article/pii/S0965229912000027

50. Zuckley L, Angelopoulou KM, Carpenter MR, McCarthy S, Meredith BA, Kline G, et al. Collagen hydrolysate improves joint function in adults with mild symptoms of osteoarthritis of the knee. Medicine & Science in Sports & Exercise. 2004;36(5):S153–4.

51. Benito-Ruiz P, Camacho-Zambrano MM, Carrillo-Arcentales JN, Mestanza-Peralta MA, Vallejo-Flores CA, Vargas-López SV, et al. A randomized controlled trial on the efficacy and safety of a food ingredient, collagen hydrolysate, for improving joint comfort. International Journal of Food Sciences and Nutrition [Internet]. 2009 Jan 1;60(sup2):99–113. Available from: https://doi.org/10.1080/09637480802498820

52. Clark KL, Sebastianelli W, Flechsenhar KR, Aukermann DF, Meza F, Millard RL, et al. 24-Week study on the use of collagen hydrolysate as a dietary supplement in athletes with activity-related joint pain. Current Medical Research and Opinion [Internet]. 2008 May 1;24(5):1485–96. Available from: https://doi.org/10.1185/030079908X291967

53. Nagaoka I. Cartilage Metabolism in Endurance Athletes and Chondroprotective Action of Glucosamine. 順天堂醫事雑誌 [Internet]. 2019;65(2):184–93. Available from: http://dx.doi.org/10.14789/jmj.2019.65.JMJ19-LN01

54. Nagaoka I. Joint Health of Athletes and the Chondroprotective Action of Glucosamine. 順天堂醫事雑誌 [Internet]. 2017;63(2):104–14. Available from: http://dx.doi.org/10.14789/jmj.63.104

55. Nagaoka I, Tsuruta A, Yoshimura M. Chondroprotective action of glucosamine, a chitosan monomer, on the joint health of athletes. International Journal of Biological Macromolecules [Internet]. 2019 July 1;132:795–800. Available from: http://www.sciencedirect.com/science/article/pii/S014181301836536X

56. Eraslan A, Ulkar B. Glucosamine Supplementation after Anterior Cruciate Ligament Reconstruction in Athletes: A Randomized Placebo-controlled Trial. Research in Sports Medicine [Internet].

2015 Jan 2;23(1):14–26. Available from:
https://doi.org/10.1080/15438627.2014.975809

57. Ostojic SM, Arsic M, Prodanovic S, Vukovic J, Zlatanovic M.
     Glucosamine Administration in Athletes: Effects on Recovery of
     Acute Knee Injury. Research in Sports Medicine [Internet]. 2007
     June 14;15(2):113–24. Available from:
     https://doi.org/10.1080/15438620701405248

58. Treede RD, Rief W, Barke A, Aziz Q, Bennett MI, Benoliel R, et al.
     A classification of chronic pain for ICD-11. PAIN [Internet].
     2015;156(6):1003–7. Available from:
     https://journals.lww.com/pain/Fulltext/2015/06000/A_classificati
     on_of_chronic_pain_for_ICD_11.6.aspx

59. Sarno JE. Etiology of neck and back pain. An automatic
     myoneuralgia? The Journal of nervous and mental disease
     [Internet]. 1981 Jan;169(1):55–9. Available from:
     https://doi.org/10.1097/00005053-198101000-00008

60. Piercy KL, Troiano RP. Physical Activity Guidelines for Americans
     From the US Department of Health and Human Services.
     Circulation: Cardiovascular Quality and Outcomes [Internet].
     2018;11(11):e005263. Available from:
     https://www.ahajournals.org/doi/abs/10.1161/CIRCOUTCOMES.
     118.005263

61. Berteus Forslund H, Torgerson JS, Sjostrom L, Lindroos AK.
     Snacking frequency in relation to energy intake and food
     choices in obese men and women compared to a reference
     population. Int J Obes Relat Metab Disord [Internet].
     2005;29(6):711–9. Available from:
     http://dx.doi.org/10.1038/sj.ijo.0802950

62. Dunn CG, Turner-McGrievy GM, Wilcox S, Hutto B. Dietary Self-Monitoring Through Calorie Tracking but Not Through a Digital Photography App Is Associated with Significant Weight Loss: The 2SMART Pilot Study—A 6-Month Randomized Trial. Journal of the Academy of Nutrition and Dietetics [Internet]. 2019 Sept 1;119(9):1525–32. Available from: https://www.sciencedirect.com/science/article/pii/S2212267219302667

63. Simpson CC, Mazzeo SE. Calorie counting and fitness tracking technology: Associations with eating disorder symptomatology. Eating Behaviors [Internet]. 2017 Aug 1;26:89–92. Available from: https://www.sciencedirect.com/science/article/pii/S1471015316303646

64. Halton TL, Hu FB. The Effects of High Protein Diets on Thermogenesis, Satiety and Weight Loss: A Critical Review. Journal of the American College of Nutrition [Internet]. 2004 Oct 1;23(5):373–85. Available from: http://dx.doi.org/10.1080/07315724.2004.10719381

65. Ortinau LC, Hoertel HA, Douglas SM, Leidy HJ. The impact of a protein-rich breakfast on food cravings and reward in overweight/obese 'breakfast skipping' adolescent girls. The FASEB Journal [Internet]. 2013;27(1_supplement):1075.9-1075.9. Available from: https://www.fasebj.org/doi/abs/10.1096/fasebj.27.1_supplement.1075.9

66. Horne BD, Muhlestein JB, Anderson JL. Health effects of intermittent fasting: hormesis or harm? A systematic review. The American Journal of Clinical Nutrition [Internet]. 2015;102(2):464–70. Available from: https://doi.org/10.3945/ajcn.115.109553

67. Derakhshan M, Derakhshan R. Fasting and Apoptosis: A Mini Review. Journal of Nutrition,Fasting and Health [Internet]. 2015;3(4):166–8. Available from: http://jnfh.mums.ac.ir/article_6314_c25aae79680a5a68a69d6c21dc8a99fa.pdf

68. Ahmed A, Saeed F, Arshad MU, Afzaal M, Imran A, Ali SW, et al. Impact of intermittent fasting on human health: an extended review of metabolic cascades. International Journal of Food Properties [Internet]. 2018 Jan 1;21(1):2700–13. Available from: https://doi.org/10.1080/10942912.2018.1560312

69. Hall KD, Guo J, Courville AB, Boring J, Brychta R, Chen KY, et al. Effect of a plant-based, low-fat diet versus an animal-based, ketogenic diet on ad libitum energy intake. Nature Medicine [Internet]. 2021 Feb 1;27(2):344–53. Available from: https://doi.org/10.1038/s41591-020-01209-1

70. Miller MA, Kruisbrink M, Wallace J, Ji C, Cappuccio FP. Sleep duration and incidence of obesity in infants, children, and adolescents: a systematic review and meta-analysis of prospective studies. Sleep [Internet]. 2018;41(4). Available from: https://doi.org/10.1093/sleep/zsy018

71. Wu Y, Gong Q, Zou Z, Li H, Zhang X. Short sleep duration and obesity among children: A systematic review and meta-analysis of prospective studies. Obesity Research & Clinical Practice [Internet]. 2017 Mar 1;11(2):140–50. Available from: http://www.sciencedirect.com/science/article/pii/S1871403X16300333

72. Li L, Zhang S, Huang Y, Chen K. Sleep duration and obesity in children: A systematic review and meta-analysis of prospective cohort studies. Journal of Paediatrics and Child Health

[Internet]. 2017;53(4):378–85. Available from:
https://onlinelibrary.wiley.com/doi/abs/10.1111/jpc.13434

73. Al Khatib HK, Harding SV, Darzi J, Pot GK. The effects of partial sleep deprivation on energy balance: a systematic review and meta-analysis. European Journal of Clinical Nutrition [Internet]. 2017 May 1;71(5):614–24. Available from: https://doi.org/10.1038/ejcn.2016.201

74. Ward AL, Reynolds AN, Kuroko S, Fangupo LJ, Galland BC, Taylor RW. Bidirectional associations between sleep and dietary intake in 0–5 year old children: A systematic review with evidence mapping. Sleep Medicine Reviews [Internet]. 2020 Feb 1;49:101231. Available from: http://www.sciencedirect.com/science/article/pii/S10870792193 01996

75. Córdova FV, Barja S, Brockmann PE. Consequences of short sleep duration on the dietary intake in children: A systematic review and metanalysis. Sleep Medicine Reviews [Internet]. 2018 Dec 1;42:68–84. Available from: http://www.sciencedirect.com/science/article/pii/S10870792173 01946

76. Geiker NRW, Astrup A, Hjorth MF, Sjödin A, Pijls L, Markus CR. Does stress influence sleep patterns, food intake, weight gain, abdominal obesity and weight loss interventions and vice versa? Obesity Reviews [Internet]. 2018;19(1):81–97. Available from: https://onlinelibrary.wiley.com/doi/abs/10.1111/obr.12603

77. Ilaria D, Elena G. Stress-Related Weight Gain: Mechanisms Involving Feeding Behavior, Metabolism, Gut Microbiota and Inflammation. Nutrition & Food Sciences. 2015;

78. Kivimäki M, Head J, Ferrie JE, Shipley MJ, Brunner E, Vahtera J, et al. Work stress, weight gain and weight loss: evidence for bidirectional effects of job strain on body mass index in the Whitehall II study. International Journal of Obesity [Internet]. 2006 June 1;30(6):982–7. Available from: https://doi.org/10.1038/sj.ijo.0803229

79. Pittas AG, Das SK, Hajduk CL, Golden J, Saltzman E, Stark PC, et al. A low-glycemic load diet facilitates greater weight loss in overweight adults with high insulin secretion but not in overweight adults with low insulin secretion in the CALERIE Trial. Diabetes Care. 2005;28(12):2939–41.

80. Cornier MA, Donahoo WT, Pereira R, Gurevich I, Westergren R, Enerback S, et al. Insulin sensitivity determines the effectiveness of dietary macronutrient composition on weight loss in obese women. Obes Res [Internet]. 2005;13(4):703–9. Available from: http://dx.doi.org/10.1038/oby.2005.79

81. Ebbeling CB, Leidig MM, Feldman HA, Lovesky MM, Ludwig DS. Effects of a low-glycemic load vs low-fat diet in obese young adults: a randomized trial. JAMA [Internet]. 2007;297(19):2092–102. Available from: http://dx.doi.org/10.1001/jama.297.19.2092

82. Le T, Flatt SW, Natarajan L, Pakiz B, Quintana EL, Heath DD, et al. Effects of diet composition and insulin resistance status on plasma lipid levels in a weight loss intervention in women. J Am Heart Assoc [Internet]. 2016;5(1). Available from: http://jaha.ahajournals.org/content/ahaoa/5/1/e002771.full.pdf

83. Gardner CD, Offringa LC, Hartle JC, Kapphahn K, Cherin R. Weight loss on low-fat vs. low-carbohydrate diets by insulin resistance status among overweight adults and adults with obesity: A randomized pilot trial. Obesity [Internet].

2016;24(1):79–86. Available from:
http://dx.doi.org/10.1002/oby.21331

84. van Erpecum CPL, van Zon SKR, Bültmann U, Smidt N. The association between fast-food outlet proximity and density and Body Mass Index: Findings from 147,027 Lifelines Cohort Study participants. Prev Med [Internet]. 2022 Feb;155:106915. Available from: http://dx.doi.org/10.1016/j.ypmed.2021.106915

85. Han J, Schwartz AE, Elbel B. Does Proximity to Fast Food Cause Childhood Obesity? Evidence from Public Housing. Reg Sci Urban Econ [Internet]. 2020 Sept;84. Available from: http://dx.doi.org/10.1016/j.regsciurbeco.2020.103565

86. Libuy N, Church D, Ploubidis G, Fitzsimons E. Fast food proximity and weight gain in childhood and adolescence: Evidence from Great Britain. Health Econ [Internet]. 2024 Mar;33(3):449–65. Available from: http://dx.doi.org/10.1002/hec.4770

87. Smagge BA, van der Velde LA, Kiefte-de Jong JC. The Food Environment Around Primary Schools in a Diverse Urban Area in the Netherlands: Linking Fast-Food Density and Proximity to Neighbourhood Disadvantage and Childhood Overweight Prevalence. Front Public Health [Internet]. 2022 Apr 6;10:838355. Available from: http://dx.doi.org/10.3389/fpubh.2022.838355

88. Woodruff RC, Haardörfer R, Raskind IG, Hermstad A, Kegler MC. Comparing food desert residents with non-food desert residents on grocery shopping behaviours, diet and BMI: results from a propensity score analysis. Public Health Nutr [Internet]. 2020 Apr;23(5):806–11. Available from: http://dx.doi.org/10.1017/S136898001900363X

89. Baxter C, Park YM. Food Swamp Versus Food Desert: Analysis of Geographic Disparities in Obesity and Diabetes in North Carolina Using GIS and Spatial Regression. Prof Geogr [Internet]. :1–16. Available from: https://doi.org/10.1080/00330124.2024.2306642

90. Larson N, Laska MN, Neumark-Sztainer D. Food Insecurity, Diet Quality, Home Food Availability, and Health Risk Behaviors Among Emerging Adults: Findings From the EAT 2010-2018 Study. Am J Public Health [Internet]. 2020 Sept;110(9):1422–8. Available from: http://dx.doi.org/10.2105/AJPH.2020.305783

91. Wolfson JA, Posluszny H, Kronsteiner-Gicevic S, Willett W, Leung CW. Food Insecurity and Less Frequent Cooking Dinner at Home Are Associated with Lower Diet Quality in a National Sample of Low-Income Adults in the United States during the Initial Months of the Coronavirus Disease 2019 Pandemic. J Acad Nutr Diet [Internet]. 2022 Oct;122(10):1893-1902.e12. Available from: http://dx.doi.org/10.1016/j.jand.2022.05.009

92. Shi Y, Grech A, Allman-Farinelli M. Diet Quality among Students Attending an Australian University Is Compromised by Food Insecurity and Less Frequent Intake of Home Cooked Meals. A Cross-Sectional Survey Using the Validated Healthy Eating Index for Australian Adults (HEIFA-2013). Nutrients [Internet]. 2022 Oct 27;14(21). Available from: http://dx.doi.org/10.3390/nu14214522

93. Clifford Astbury C, Penney TL, Adams J. Home-prepared food, dietary quality and socio-demographic factors: a cross-sectional analysis of the UK National Diet and nutrition survey 2008-16. Int J Behav Nutr Phys Act [Internet]. 2019 Sept 6;16(1):82. Available from: http://dx.doi.org/10.1186/s12966-019-0846-x

94. Rex SM, Kopetsky A, Bodt B, Robson SM. Relationships Among the Physical and Social Home Food Environments, Dietary Intake, and Diet Quality in Mothers and Children. J Acad Nutr Diet [Internet]. 2021 Oct;121(10):2013-2020.e1. Available from: http://dx.doi.org/10.1016/j.jand.2021.03.008

95. Qiu N, Moore JB, Wang Y, Fu J, Ding K, Li R. Perceived Parental Attitudes Are Indirectly Associated with Consumption of Junk Foods and Sugar-Sweetened Beverages among Chinese Adolescents through Home Food Environment and Autonomous Motivation: A Path Analysis. Nutrients [Internet]. 2021 Sept 27;13(10). Available from: http://dx.doi.org/10.3390/nu13103403

96. Ortega-Avila AG, Papadaki A, Jago R. The role of the home environment in sugar-sweetened beverage intake among northern Mexican adolescents: a qualitative study. J Public Health [Internet]. 2019 Dec 1;27(6):791–801. Available from: https://doi.org/10.1007/s10389-018-0993-6

97. Bassul C, A Corish C, M Kearney J. Associations between the Home Environment, Feeding Practices and Children's Intakes of Fruit, Vegetables and Confectionary/Sugar-Sweetened Beverages. Int J Environ Res Public Health [Internet]. 2020 July 5;17(13). Available from: http://dx.doi.org/10.3390/ijerph17134837

98. Baghlaf K, Muirhead V, Pine C. Relationships between children's sugar consumption at home and their food choices and consumption at school lunch. Public Health Nutr [Internet]. 2020 Nov;23(16):2941–9. Available from: http://dx.doi.org/10.1017/S1368980019003458

99. Zhao J, Stockwell T, Naimi T, Churchill S, Clay J, Sherk A. Association between daily alcohol intake and risk of all-cause

mortality: A systematic review and meta-analyses: A systematic review and meta-analyses. JAMA Netw Open [Internet]. 2023 Mar 1 [cited 2025 Feb 25];6(3):e236185. Available from: https://jamanetwork.com/journals/jamanetworkopen/articlepdf/2802963/zhao_2023_oi_230209_1683218447.95134.pdf

100. Zhu JZ, Wang YM, Zhou QY, Zhu KF, Yu CH, Li YM. Systematic review with meta-analysis: alcohol consumption and the risk of colorectal adenoma. Alimentary Pharmacology & Therapeutics [Internet]. 2014;40(4):325–37. Available from: http://search.ebscohost.com/login.aspx?direct=true&db=mdc&AN=24943329&site=ehost-live

101. Taylor B, Rehm J, Gmel G. Moderate alcohol consumption and the gastrointestinal tract. Digestive Diseases (Basel, Switzerland) [Internet]. 2005;23(3–4):170–6. Available from: http://search.ebscohost.com/login.aspx?direct=true&db=mdc&AN=16508280&site=ehost-live

102. Mostofsky E, Lee IM, Buring JE, Mukamal KJ. Impact of alcohol consumption on breast cancer incidence and mortality: The women's health study. J Womens Health (Larchmt) [Internet]. 2024 June 13 [cited 2024 July 4];33(6):705–14. Available from: https://www.liebertpub.com/doi/10.1089/jwh.2023.1021

103. Li Q, Liu Y, Sun X, Yin Z, Li H, Cheng C, et al. Caffeinated and decaffeinated coffee consumption and risk of all-cause mortality: a dose-response meta-analysis of cohort studies. J Hum Nutr Diet [Internet]. 2019 June 1 [cited 2025 Oct 16];32(3):279–87. Available from: http://dx.doi.org/10.1111/jhn.12633

104. Kim Y, Je Y, Giovannucci E. Coffee consumption and all-cause and cause-specific mortality: a meta-analysis by potential modifiers. Eur J Epidemiol [Internet]. 2019 Aug 4 [cited 2025 Oct

16];34(8):731–52. Available from:
http://dx.doi.org/10.1007/s10654-019-00524-3

105.   Fatolahi H, Farahmand A, Rezakhani S. The Effect of Caffeine on Health and Exercise Performance with a Cold Brew Coffee Approach: A Scoping Review. Nutrition and Food Sciences Research. 2020;7(2):1–12.

106.   Astorino TA, Roberson DW. Efficacy of Acute Caffeine Ingestion for Short-term High-Intensity Exercise Performance: A Systematic Review. The Journal of Strength & Conditioning Research [Internet]. 2010;24(1):257–65. Available from: https://journals.lww.com/nsca-jscr/Fulltext/2010/01000/Efficacy_of_Acute_Caffeine_Ingestion_for.38.aspx

107.   Grgic J, Mikulic P, Schoenfeld BJ, Bishop DJ, Pedisic Z. The Influence of Caffeine Supplementation on Resistance Exercise: A Review. Sports Medicine [Internet]. 2019 Jan 1;49(1):17–30. Available from: https://doi.org/10.1007/s40279-018-0997-y

108.   Southward K, Rutherfurd-Markwick KJ, Ali A. The Effect of Acute Caffeine Ingestion on Endurance Performance: A Systematic Review and Meta–Analysis. Sports Medicine [Internet]. 2018 Aug 1;48(8):1913–28. Available from: https://doi.org/10.1007/s40279-018-0939-8

109.   Grgic J, Grgic I, Pickering C, Schoenfeld BJ, Bishop DJ, Pedisic Z. Wake up and smell the coffee: caffeine supplementation and exercise performance—an umbrella review of 21 published meta-analyses. British Journal of Sports Medicine [Internet]. 2020;54(11):681–8. Available from: https://bjsm.bmj.com/content/bjsports/54/11/681.full.pdf

110.   Polito MD, Souza DB, Casonatto J, Farinatti P. Acute effect of caffeine consumption on isotonic muscular strength and endurance: A systematic review and meta-analysis. Science & Sports [Internet]. 2016 June 1;31(3):119–28. Available from: http://www.sciencedirect.com/science/article/pii/S0765159716000563

111.   Crawford C, Teo L, Lafferty L, Drake A, Bingham JJ, Gallon MD, et al. Caffeine to optimize cognitive function for military mission-readiness: a systematic review and recommendations for the field. Nutrition Reviews [Internet]. 2017;75(suppl_2):17–35. Available from: https://doi.org/10.1093/nutrit/nux007

112.   Irwin C, Khalesi S, Desbrow B, McCartney D. Effects of acute caffeine consumption following sleep loss on cognitive, physical, occupational and driving performance: A systematic review and meta-analysis. Neuroscience & Biobehavioral Reviews [Internet]. 2020 Jan 1;108:877–88. Available from: http://www.sciencedirect.com/science/article/pii/S0149763419307377

113.   Ruxton CHS. The impact of caffeine on mood, cognitive function, performance and hydration: a review of benefits and risks. Nutrition Bulletin [Internet]. 2008;33(1):15–25. Available from: https://onlinelibrary.wiley.com/doi/abs/10.1111/j.1467-3010.2007.00665.x

114.   Cheung HTH. Impact of caffeine on macronutrient metabolism: A review of literature. 2016;

115.   Schubert MM, Irwin C, Seay RF, Clarke HE, Allegro D, Desbrow B. Caffeine, coffee, and appetite control: a review. International Journal of Food Sciences and Nutrition [Internet]. 2017 Nov 17;68(8):901–12. Available from: https://doi.org/10.1080/09637486.2017.1320537

116.　Lazou E, Vlastos I, Gkouskou K, Skoufas E, Chaniotis D. Coffee intake reduces short-term carbohydrate and lipid consumption. Dietetics [Internet]. 2025 May 12 [cited 2025 May 16];4(2):20. Available from: http://dx.doi.org/10.3390/dietetics4020020

117.　吳柏翰. Timing effects of caffeine ingestion on acute testosterone and cortisol responses to resistance exercise. 體育學報 [Internet]. 2019;52(S):31–45. Available from: http://dx.doi.org/10.3966/10247297201903520s003

118.　Yaghoubi A, Davoudi M, Taheri Chadorneshin H. The Eeffect of Caffeine Ingestion on Cortisol and Some Immune Factors Response to Exhaustive Exercise in Inactive Women. Journal of Sport Biosciences [Internet]. 2017;8(4):591–606. Available from: https://jsb.ut.ac.ir/article_61243_7501b1d196d18d1cbef991d57646bf70.pdf

119.　Beaven CM, Hopkins WG, Hansen KT, Wood MR, Cronin JB, Lowe TE. Dose Effect of Caffeine on Testosterone and Cortisol Responses to Resistance Exercise. International Journal of Sport Nutrition and Exercise Metabolism [Internet]. 2008 Apr 1;18(2):131–41. Available from: https://journals.humankinetics.com/view/journals/ijsnem/18/2/article-p131.xml

120.　Hirshkowitz M, Whiton K, Albert SM, Alessi C, Bruni O, DonCarlos L, et al. National Sleep Foundation's sleep time duration recommendations: methodology and results summary. Sleep Health: Journal of the National Sleep Foundation [Internet]. 1(1):40–3. Available from: http://dx.doi.org/10.1016/j.sleh.2014.12.010

121.　Altevogt BM, Colten HR. Sleep disorders and sleep deprivation: an unmet public health problem. National Academies Press; 2006.

244

122.   Anothaisintawee T, Reutrakul S, Van Cauter E, Thakkinstian A. Sleep disturbances compared to traditional risk factors for diabetes development: Systematic review and meta-analysis. Sleep Medicine Reviews [Internet]. 2016 Dec 1;30:11–24. Available from: http://www.sciencedirect.com/science/article/pii/S10870792150 0146X

123.   Lee SWH, Ng KY, Chin WK. The impact of sleep amount and sleep quality on glycemic control in type 2 diabetes: A systematic review and meta-analysis. Sleep Medicine Reviews [Internet]. 2017 Feb 1;31:91–101. Available from: http://www.sciencedirect.com/science/article/pii/S10870792160 00174

124.   Itani O, Jike M, Watanabe N, Kaneita Y. Short sleep duration and health outcomes: a systematic review, meta-analysis, and meta-regression. Sleep Medicine [Internet]. 2017 Apr 1;32:246–56. Available from: http://www.sciencedirect.com/science/article/pii/S13899457163 01381

125.   Silva AA da, Mello RGB de, Schaan CW, Fuchs FD, Redline S, Fuchs SC. Sleep duration and mortality in the elderly: a systematic review with meta-analysis. BMJ Open [Internet]. 2016;6(2):e008119. Available from: https://bmjopen.bmj.com/content/bmjopen/6/2/e008119.full.p df

126.   Jike M, Itani O, Watanabe N, Buysse DJ, Kaneita Y. Long sleep duration and health outcomes: A systematic review, meta-analysis and meta-regression. Sleep Medicine Reviews [Internet]. 2018 June 1;39:25–36. Available from: http://www.sciencedirect.com/science/article/pii/S10870792173 00278

127.   Yin J, Jin X, Shan Z, Li S, Huang H, Li P, et al. Relationship of Sleep Duration With All-Cause Mortality and Cardiovascular Events: A Systematic Review and Dose-Response Meta-Analysis of Prospective Cohort Studies. Journal of the American Heart Association [Internet]. 2017;6(9):e005947. Available from: https://www.ahajournals.org/doi/abs/10.1161/JAHA.117.005947

128.   Gottlieb E, Landau E, Baxter H, Werden E, Howard ME, Brodtmann A. The bidirectional impact of sleep and circadian rhythm dysfunction in human ischaemic stroke: A systematic review. Sleep Medicine Reviews [Internet]. 2019 June 1;45:54–69. Available from: http://www.sciencedirect.com/science/article/pii/S1087079218300856

129.   Leong RLF, Cheng GHL, Chee MWL, Lo JC. The effects of sleep on prospective memory: A systematic review and meta-analysis. Sleep Medicine Reviews [Internet]. 2019 Oct 1;47:18–27. Available from: http://www.sciencedirect.com/science/article/pii/S1087079219300140

130.   Lo JC, Groeger JA, Cheng GH, Dijk DJ, Chee MWL. Self-reported sleep duration and cognitive performance in older adults: a systematic review and meta-analysis. Sleep Medicine [Internet]. 2016 Jan 1;17:87–98. Available from: http://www.sciencedirect.com/science/article/pii/S1389945715019796

131.   Leng Y, McEvoy CT, Allen IE, Yaffe K. Association of Sleep-Disordered Breathing With Cognitive Function and Risk of Cognitive Impairment: A Systematic Review and Meta-analysis. JAMA Neurology [Internet]. 2017;74(10):1237–45. Available from: https://doi.org/10.1001/jamaneurol.2017.2180

132.   Bubu OM, Brannick M, Mortimer J, Umasabor-Bubu O, Sebastião YV, Wen Y, et al. Sleep, Cognitive impairment, and Alzheimer's disease: A Systematic Review and Meta-Analysis. Sleep [Internet]. 2016;40(1). Available from: https://doi.org/10.1093/sleep/zsw032

133.   Konjarski M, Murray G, Lee VV, Jackson ML. Reciprocal relationships between daily sleep and mood: A systematic review of naturalistic prospective studies. Sleep Medicine Reviews [Internet]. 2018 Dec 1;42:47–58. Available from: http://www.sciencedirect.com/science/article/pii/S10870792173 01582

134.   Cox RC, Olatunji BO. A systematic review of sleep disturbance in anxiety and related disorders. Journal of Anxiety Disorders [Internet]. 2016 Jan 1;37:104–29. Available from: http://www.sciencedirect.com/science/article/pii/S08876185153 00384

135.   Pires GN, Bezerra AG, Tufik S, Andersen ML. Effects of acute sleep deprivation on state anxiety levels: a systematic review and meta-analysis. Sleep Medicine [Internet]. 2016 Aug 1;24:109–18. Available from: http://www.sciencedirect.com/science/article/pii/S13899457163 01368

136.   Bao YP, Han Y, Ma J, Wang RJ, Shi L, Wang TY, et al. Cooccurrence and bidirectional prediction of sleep disturbances and depression in older adults: Meta-analysis and systematic review. Neuroscience & Biobehavioral Reviews [Internet]. 2017 Apr 1;75:257–73. Available from: http://www.sciencedirect.com/science/article/pii/S01497634163 05097

137.   Galbiati A, Verga L, Giora E, Zucconi M, Ferini-Strambi L. The risk of neurodegeneration in REM sleep behavior disorder: A systematic review and meta-analysis of longitudinal studies. Sleep Medicine Reviews [Internet]. 2019 Feb 1;43:37–46. Available from: http://www.sciencedirect.com/science/article/pii/S1087079218300819

138.   Campanini MZ, Guallar-Castillón P, Rodríguez-Artalejo F, Lopez-Garcia E. Mediterranean Diet and Changes in Sleep Duration and Indicators of Sleep Quality in Older Adults. Sleep [Internet]. 2016;40(3). Available from: https://doi.org/10.1093/sleep/zsw083

139.   Godos J, Ferri R, Caraci F, Cosentino FII, Castellano S, Galvano F, et al. Adherence to the Mediterranean Diet is Associated with Better Sleep Quality in Italian Adults. Nutrients [Internet]. 2019;11(5):976. Available from: https://www.mdpi.com/2072-6643/11/5/976

140.   Mamalaki E, Anastasiou CA, Ntanasi E, Tsapanou A, Kosmidis MH, Dardiotis E, et al. Associations between the mediterranean diet and sleep in older adults: Results from the hellenic longitudinal investigation of aging and diet study. Geriatrics & Gerontology International [Internet]. 2018;18(11):1543–8. Available from: https://onlinelibrary.wiley.com/doi/abs/10.1111/ggi.13521

141.   Ferranti R, Marventano S, Castellano S, Giogianni G, Nolfo F, Rametta S, et al. Sleep quality and duration is related with diet and obesity in young adolescent living in Sicily, Southern Italy. Sleep Science [Internet]. 2016 Apr 1;9(2):117–22. Available from: http://www.sciencedirect.com/science/article/pii/S1984006316300049

142.   Pagliai G, Dinu M, Casini A, Sofi F. Relationship between sleep pattern and efficacy of calorie-restricted Mediterranean diet in overweight/obese subjects. International Journal of Food Sciences and Nutrition [Internet]. 2018 Jan 2;69(1):93–9. Available from: https://doi.org/10.1080/09637486.2017.1330405

143.   Letellier LR. Sleep duration and its association with diet quality and weight status [Internet]. The Ohio State University; 2019. Available from: http://rave.ohiolink.edu/etdc/view?acc_num=osu1555430762220235

144.   St-Onge MP, Mikic A, Pietrolungo CE. Effects of Diet on Sleep Quality. Advances in Nutrition [Internet]. 2016;7(5):938–49. Available from: https://doi.org/10.3945/an.116.012336

145.   Zuraikat FM, St-Onge MP. Chapter 22 - The Influence of Diet on Sleep. In: Watson RR, Preedy VR, editors. Neurological Modulation of Sleep [Internet]. Academic Press; 2020. p. 205–15. Available from: http://www.sciencedirect.com/science/article/pii/B9780128166581000223

146.   Noorwali EA, Cade JE, Burley VJ, Hardie LJ. The relationship between sleep duration and fruit/vegetable intakes in UK adults: a cross-sectional study from the National Diet and Nutrition Survey. BMJ Open [Internet]. 2018;8(4):e020810. Available from: http://bmjopen.bmj.com/content/8/4/e020810.abstract

147.   Burgess V, Carson C, Ellerbroek A, Axelrod C, Peacock C, Silver TA, et al. High-Protein Diet has no Effect on Sleep Quality and Quantity in Exercise-Trained Men and Women. Journal of Exercise and Nutrition. 2019;2(1):1.

148.   Metlaine A. Chapter 25 - Sleep, Stress, and Vitamin D. In: Watson RR, Preedy VR, editors. Neurological Modulation of Sleep [Internet]. Academic Press; 2020. p. 235–42. Available from: http://www.sciencedirect.com/science/article/pii/B97801281665 81000259

149.   van Maanen A, Meijer AM, van der Heijden KB, Oort FJ. The effects of light therapy on sleep problems: A systematic review and meta-analysis. Sleep Medicine Reviews [Internet]. 2016 Oct 1;29:52–62. Available from: http://www.sciencedirect.com/science/article/pii/S10870792150 01136

150.   He M, Ru T, Li S, Li Y, Zhou G. Shine light on sleep: Morning bright light improves nocturnal sleep and next morning alertness among college students. J Sleep Res [Internet]. 2023 Apr 1 [cited 2025 Oct 1];32(2):e13724. Available from: http://dx.doi.org/10.1111/jsr.13724

151.   Amdisen L, Daugaard S, Vestergaard JM, Vested A, Bonde JP, Vistisen HT, et al. A longitudinal study of morning, evening, and night light intensities and nocturnal sleep quality in a working population. Chronobiol Int [Internet]. 2022 Apr [cited 2025 Oct 1];39(4):579–89. Available from: http://dx.doi.org/10.1080/07420528.2021.2010741

152.   Muscogiuri G, Barrea L, Scannapieco M, Di Somma C, Scacchi M, Aimaretti G, et al. The lullaby of the sun: the role of vitamin D in sleep disturbance. Sleep Medicine [Internet]. 2019 Feb 1;54:262–5. Available from: http://www.sciencedirect.com/science/article/pii/S13899457183 06014

153. Mohammad Shahi M, Hosseini SA, Helli B, Haghighyzade MH, Abolfathi M. The effect of vitamin D supplement on quality of sleep in adult people with sleep disorders. Tehran University Medical Journal [Internet]. 2017;75(6):443–8. Available from: http://tumj.tums.ac.ir/article-1-8272-en.html

154. Gao Q, Kou T, Zhuang B, Ren Y, Dong X, Wang Q. The Association between Vitamin D Deficiency and Sleep Disorders: A Systematic Review and Meta-Analysis. Nutrients [Internet]. 2018;10(10):1395. Available from: https://www.mdpi.com/2072-6643/10/10/1395

155. Murck H, Holsboer F, Steiger A. Magnesium sulphate has GABA-Agonistic effects on sleep in healthy men. Biological Psychiatry [Internet]. 1996;39(7):591. Available from: https://doi.org/10.1016/0006-3223(96)84257-0

156. Murck H, Held K, Auer DP, Steiger A. Therapeutic sleep deprivation and magnesium: Modulators of the GABA/glutamate equilibrium. Pharmacopsychiatry [Internet]. 2003;36(05):201. Available from: http://dx.doi.org/10.1055/s-2003-825452

157. Nielsen FH. Chapter 31 - Relation between Magnesium Deficiency and Sleep Disorders and Associated Pathological Changes. In: Watson RR, editor. Modulation of Sleep by Obesity, Diabetes, Age, and Diet [Internet]. San Diego: Academic Press; 2015. p. 291–6. Available from: http://www.sciencedirect.com/science/article/pii/B978012420167 82000314

158. Dralle D, Bödeker RH. Serum magnesium level and sleep behavior of newborn infants. European Journal of Pediatrics [Internet]. 1980 Sept 1;134(3):239–43. Available from: https://doi.org/10.1007/BF00441479

159.   Takase B, Akima T, Satomura K, Fumitaka, Ohsuzu, Mastui T, et al. Effects of chronic sleep deprivation on autonomic activity by examining heart rate variability, plasma catecholamine, and intracellular magnesium levels. Biomedicine & Pharmacotherapy [Internet]. 2004 Oct 1;58:S35–9. Available from: http://www.sciencedirect.com/science/article/pii/S0753332204800076

160.   Cao Y, Zhen S, Taylor AW, Appleton S, Atlantis E, Shi Z. Magnesium Intake and Sleep Disorder Symptoms: Findings from the Jiangsu Nutrition Study of Chinese Adults at Five-Year Follow-Up. Nutrients [Internet]. 2018;10(10):1354. Available from: https://www.mdpi.com/2072-6643/10/10/1354

161.   Tanabe K, Yamamoto A, Suzuki N, Osada N, Yokoyama Y, Samejima H, et al. Efficacy of Oral Magnesium Administration on Decreased Exercise Tolerance in a State of Chronic Sleep Deprivation. JAPANESE CIRCULATION JOURNAL [Internet]. 1998;62(5):341–6. Available from: http://dx.doi.org/10.1253/jcj.62.341

162.   Nielsen FH. Magnesium supplementation improves indicators of low magnesium status and inflammatory stress in adults older than 51 years with poor quality sleep. Magnesium Research [Internet]. 2010 Dec 10;23(4):158-168–2010 v.23 no.4. Available from: http://dx.doi.org/10.1684/mrh.2010.0220

163.   Cherasse Y, Urade Y. Dietary Zinc Acts as a Sleep Modulator. International Journal of Molecular Sciences [Internet]. 2017;18(11):2334. Available from: https://www.mdpi.com/1422-0067/18/11/2334

164.   Saito H, Cherasse Y, Suzuki R, Mitarai M, Ueda F, Urade Y. Zinc-rich oysters as well as zinc-yeast- and astaxanthin-enriched

food improved sleep efficiency and sleep onset in a randomized controlled trial of healthy individuals. Molecular Nutrition & Food Research [Internet]. 2017;61(5):1600882. Available from: https://onlinelibrary.wiley.com/doi/abs/10.1002/mnfr.20160088 2

165.   Gholipour Baradari A, Alipour A, Mahdavi A, Sharifi H, Nouraei SM, Emami Zeydi A. The Effect of Zinc Supplementation on Sleep Quality of ICU Nurses: A Double Blinded Randomized Controlled Trial. Workplace Health & Safety [Internet]. 2018;66(4):191–200. Available from: https://journals.sagepub.com/doi/abs/10.1177/2165079917734 880

166.   Shallcross AJ, Visvanathan PD, Sperber SH, Duberstein ZT. Waking up to the problem of sleep: can mindfulness help? A review of theory and evidence for the effects of mindfulness for sleep. Current Opinion in Psychology [Internet]. 2019 Aug 1;28:37–41. Available from: http://www.sciencedirect.com/science/article/pii/S2352250X183 01404

167.   Winbush NY, Gross CR, Kreitzer MJ. The Effects of Mindfulness-Based Stress Reduction on Sleep Disturbance: A Systematic Review. EXPLORE [Internet]. 2007 Nov 1;3(6):585–91. Available from: http://www.sciencedirect.com/science/article/pii/S15508307070 02741

168.   Rusch HL, Rosario M, Levison LM, Olivera A, Livingston WS, Wu T, et al. The effect of mindfulness meditation on sleep quality: a systematic review and meta-analysis of randomized controlled trials. Annals of the New York Academy of Sciences [Internet]. 2019;1445(1):5–16. Available from:

253

https://nyaspubs.onlinelibrary.wiley.com/doi/abs/10.1111/nyas.
13996

169.   Wang Q, Zhang X, Wang Q, Zhang W. Interventional effect of
mindfulness-based stress reduction on perceived stress and
sleep disturbance in cancer patients: a systematic review.
Chongqing Medicine. 2017;46(25):3547–50.

170.   Wang F, Eun-Kyoung Lee O, Feng F, Vitiello MV, Wang W,
Benson H, et al. The effect of meditative movement on sleep
quality: A systematic review. Sleep Medicine Reviews [Internet].
2016 Dec 1;30:43–52. Available from:
http://www.sciencedirect.com/science/article/pii/S10870792150
01604

171.   Zeichner SB, Zeichner RL, Gogineni K, Shatil S, Ioachimescu
O. Cognitive Behavioral Therapy for Insomnia, Mindfulness, and
Yoga in Patients With Breast Cancer with Sleep Disturbance: A
Literature Review. Breast Cancer: Basic and Clinical Research
[Internet]. 2017;11:1178223417745564. Available from:
https://journals.sagepub.com/doi/abs/10.1177/1178223417745
564

172.   Zou L, Yeung A, Quan X, Boyden SD, Wang H. A Systematic
Review and Meta-Analysis of Mindfulness-Based (Baduanjin)
Exercise for Alleviating Musculoskeletal Pain and Improving
Sleep Quality in People with Chronic Diseases. International
Journal of Environmental Research and Public Health [Internet].
2018;15(2):206. Available from: https://www.mdpi.com/1660-
4601/15/2/206

173.   Bonnar D, Bartel K, Kakoschke N, Lang C. Sleep Interventions
Designed to Improve Athletic Performance and Recovery: A
Systematic Review of Current Approaches. Sports Medicine

[Internet]. 2018 Mar 1;48(3):683–703. Available from:
https://doi.org/10.1007/s40279-017-0832-x

174.   Patterson PD, Ghen JD, Antoon SF, Martin-Gill C, Guyette FX,
Weiss PM, et al. Does evidence support "banking/extending
sleep" by shift workers to mitigate fatigue, and/or to improve
health, safety, or performance? A systematic review. Sleep
Health [Internet]. 2019 Aug 1;5(4):359–69. Available from:
http://www.sciencedirect.com/science/article/pii/S23527218193
00592

175.   Haghayegh S, Khoshnevis S, Smolensky MH, Diller KR,
Castriotta RJ. Before-bedtime passive body heating by warm
shower or bath to improve sleep: A systematic review and
meta-analysis. Sleep Med Rev [Internet]. 2019;46:124–35.
Available from: http://dx.doi.org/10.1016/j.smrv.2019.04.008

176.   Kelley GA, Kelley KS. Exercise and sleep: a systematic review
of previous meta-analyses. Journal of Evidence-Based Medicine
[Internet]. 2017;10(1):26–36. Available from:
https://onlinelibrary.wiley.com/doi/abs/10.1111/jebm.12236

177.   Dolezal BA, Neufeld EV, Boland DM, Martin JL, Cooper CB.
Interrelationship between Sleep and Exercise: A Systematic
Review. Advances in Preventive Medicine [Internet]. 2017 Mar
26;2017:1364387. Available from:
https://doi.org/10.1155/2017/1364387

178.   Lederman O, Ward PB, Firth J, Maloney C, Carney R,
Vancampfort D, et al. Does exercise improve sleep quality in
individuals with mental illness? A systematic review and meta-
analysis. Journal of Psychiatric Research [Internet]. 2019 Feb
1;109:96–106. Available from:
http://www.sciencedirect.com/science/article/pii/S00223956183
08525

179. Rubio-Arias JÁ, Marín-Cascales E, Ramos-Campo DJ, Hernandez AV, Pérez-López FR. Effect of exercise on sleep quality and insomnia in middle-aged women: A systematic review and meta-analysis of randomized controlled trials. Maturitas [Internet]. 2017 June 1;100:49–56. Available from: http://www.sciencedirect.com/science/article/pii/S03785122173 04838

180. Lowe H, Haddock G, Mulligan LD, Gregg L, Fuzellier-Hart A, Carter LA, et al. Does exercise improve sleep for adults with insomnia? A systematic review with quality appraisal. Clinical Psychology Review [Internet]. 2019 Mar 1;68:1–12. Available from: http://www.sciencedirect.com/science/article/pii/S02727358173 03306

181. Stutz J, Eiholzer R, Spengler CM. Effects of Evening Exercise on Sleep in Healthy Participants: A Systematic Review and Meta-Analysis. Sports Medicine [Internet]. 2019 Feb 1;49(2):269–87. Available from: https://doi.org/10.1007/s40279-018-1015-0

182. Kovacevic A, Mavros Y, Heisz JJ, Fiatarone Singh MA. The effect of resistance exercise on sleep: A systematic review of randomized controlled trials. Sleep Medicine Reviews [Internet]. 2018 June 1;39:52–68. Available from: http://www.sciencedirect.com/science/article/pii/S10870792163 01526

183. Carter B, Rees P, Hale L, Bhattacharjee D, Paradkar MS. Association Between Portable Screen-Based Media Device Access or Use and Sleep Outcomes: A Systematic Review and Meta-analysis. JAMA Pediatrics [Internet]. 2016;170(12):1202–8. Available from: https://doi.org/10.1001/jamapediatrics.2016.2341

184.   Alimoradi Z, Lin CY, Broström A, Bülow PH, Bajalan Z, Griffiths MD, et al. Internet addiction and sleep problems: A systematic review and meta-analysis. Sleep Medicine Reviews [Internet]. 2019 Oct 1;47:51–61. Available from: http://www.sciencedirect.com/science/article/pii/S1087079219300267

185.   Panza F, Solfrizzi V, Barulli MR, Bonfiglio C, Guerra V, Osella A, et al. Coffee, tea, and caffeine consumption and prevention of late-life cognitive decline and dementia: A systematic review. The journal of nutrition, health & aging [Internet]. 2015;19(3):313–28. Available from: https://doi.org/10.1007/s12603-014-0563-8

186.   Clark I, Landolt HP. Coffee, caffeine, and sleep: A systematic review of epidemiological studies and randomized controlled trials. Sleep Medicine Reviews [Internet]. 2017 Feb 1;31:70–8. Available from: http://www.sciencedirect.com/science/article/pii/S1087079216000150

187.   Simou E, Britton J, Leonardi-Bee J. Alcohol and the risk of sleep apnoea: a systematic review and meta-analysis. Sleep Medicine [Internet]. 2018 Feb 1;42:38–46. Available from: http://www.sciencedirect.com/science/article/pii/S1389945717315988

188.   Basner M, McGuire S. WHO Environmental Noise Guidelines for the European Region: A Systematic Review on Environmental Noise and Effects on Sleep. International Journal of Environmental Research and Public Health [Internet]. 2018;15(3):519. Available from: https://www.mdpi.com/1660-4601/15/3/519

189.   van Dalfsen JH, Markus CR. The influence of sleep on human hypothalamic–pituitary–adrenal (HPA) axis reactivity: A systematic review. Sleep Medicine Reviews [Internet]. 2018 June 1;39:187–94. Available from: http://www.sciencedirect.com/science/article/pii/S10870792173 01119

190.   Friedrich A, Schlarb AA. Let's talk about sleep: a systematic review of psychological interventions to improve sleep in college students. Journal of Sleep Research [Internet]. 2018;27(1):4–22. Available from: https://onlinelibrary.wiley.com/doi/abs/10.1111/jsr.12568

191.   Mitchell LJ, Bisdounis L, Ballesio A, Omlin X, Kyle SD. The impact of cognitive behavioural therapy for insomnia on objective sleep parameters: A meta-analysis and systematic review. Sleep Medicine Reviews [Internet]. 2019 Oct 1;47:90–102. Available from: http://www.sciencedirect.com/science/article/pii/S10870792183 02223

192.   Shields GS, Slavich GM. Lifetime stress exposure and health: A review of contemporary assessment methods and biological mechanisms. Social and Personality Psychology Compass [Internet]. 2017 Aug 1;11(8):e12335. Available from: https://doi.org/10.1111/spc3.12335

193.   Costa B, Pinto IC. Stress, burnout and coping in health professionals: a literature review. Journal of Psychology and Brain Studies. 2017;1(1: 4):1–8.

194.   Verkuil B, Brosschot JF, Gebhardt WA, Thayer JF. When Worries Make you Sick: A Review of Perseverative Cognition, the Default Stress Response and Somatic Health. Journal of Experimental Psychopathology [Internet]. 2010;1(1):jep.009110.

Available from:
https://journals.sagepub.com/doi/abs/10.5127/jep.009110

195.   Slavich GM. Life Stress and Health:A Review of Conceptual
        Issues and Recent Findings. Teaching of Psychology [Internet].
        2016;43(4):346–55. Available from:
        https://journals.sagepub.com/doi/abs/10.1177/0098628316662
        768

196.   de Boer J, Lok A, van't Verlaat E, Duivenvoorden HJ, Bakker
        AB, Smit BJ. Work-related critical incidents in hospital-based
        health care providers and the risk of post-traumatic stress
        symptoms, anxiety, and depression: A meta-analysis. Social
        Science & Medicine [Internet]. 2011 July 1;73(2):316–26.
        Available from:
        http://www.sciencedirect.com/science/article/pii/S02779536110
        02838

197.   Sachs-Ericsson N, Cromer K, Hernandez A, Kendall-Tackett K.
        A Review of Childhood Abuse, Health, and Pain-Related
        Problems: The Role of Psychiatric Disorders and Current Life
        Stress. Journal of Trauma & Dissociation [Internet]. 2009 Apr
        3;10(2):170–88. Available from:
        https://doi.org/10.1080/15299730802624585

198.   Garfin DR, Thompson RR, Holman EA. Acute stress and
        subsequent health outcomes: A systematic review. Journal of
        Psychosomatic Research [Internet]. 2018 Sept 1;112:107–13.
        Available from:
        http://www.sciencedirect.com/science/article/pii/S00223999183
        00692

199.   Turner AI, Smyth N, Hall SJ, Torres SJ, Hussein M, Jayasinghe
        SU, et al. Psychological stress reactivity and future health and
        disease outcomes: A systematic review of prospective evidence.

Psychoneuroendocrinology [Internet]. 2020 Apr 1;114:104599. Available from: http://www.sciencedirect.com/science/article/pii/S03064530203 00184

200.   Eddy P, Wertheim EH, Kingsley M, Wright BJ. Associations between the effort-reward imbalance model of workplace stress and indices of cardiovascular health: A systematic review and meta-analysis. Neuroscience & Biobehavioral Reviews [Internet]. 2017 Dec 1;83:252–66. Available from: http://www.sciencedirect.com/science/article/pii/S01497634173 0458X

201.   Kim J, Kim HR. The relationship between increased job stress and weight gain: a 2-year longitudinal study. Occupational and Environmental Medicine [Internet]. 2011;68(Suppl 1):A76–7. Available from: https://oem.bmj.com/content/oemed/68/Suppl_1/A76.4.full.pdf

202.   Klingberg S, Mehlig K, Johansson I, Lindahl B, Winkvist A, Lissner L. Occupational stress is associated with major long-term weight gain in a Swedish population-based cohort. International archives of occupational and environmental health. 2019;92(4):569–76.

203.   Berset M, Semmer NK, Elfering A, Jacobshagen N, Meier LL. Does stress at work make you gain weight? A two-year longitudinal study. Scandinavian Journal of Work, Environment & Health [Internet]. 2011;37(1):45–53. Available from: http://www.jstor.org/stable/40967886

204.   Fincham GW, Mavor K, Dritschel B. Effects of mindfulness meditation duration and type on well-being: An online dose-ranging randomized controlled trial. Mindfulness (N Y) [Internet]. 2023 Apr 12 [cited 2024 Oct 15];14(5):1171–82.

Available from:
https://link.springer.com/article/10.1007/s12671-023-02119-2

205.   Strohmaier S. The relationship between doses of
        mindfulness-based programs and depression, anxiety, stress,
        and mindfulness: A dose-response meta-regression of
        randomized controlled trials. Mindfulness (N Y) [Internet]. 2020
        June 2 [cited 2024 Oct 15];11(6):1315–35. Available from:
        https://link.springer.com/article/10.1007/s12671-020-01319-4

206.   Levi K, Shoham A, Amir I, Bernstein A. The daily dose-
        response hypothesis of mindfulness meditation practice: An
        experience sampling study: An experience sampling study.
        Psychosom Med [Internet]. 2021 [cited 2024 Oct 15];83(6):624–
        30. Available from:
        https://journals.lww.com/psychosomaticmedicine/abstract/202
        1/07000/the_daily_dose_response_hypothesis_of_mindfulness.1
        4.aspx

207.   Cearns M, Clark SR. The effects of dose, practice habits, and
        objects of focus on digital meditation effectiveness and
        adherence: Longitudinal study of 280,000 digital meditation
        sessions across 103 countries. J Med Internet Res [Internet].
        2023 Sept 19 [cited 2024 Oct 15];25(1):e43358. Available from:
        https://www.jmir.org/2023/1/e43358

www.ingramcontent.com/pod-product-compliance
Lightning Source LLC
Chambersburg PA
CBHW051256020426
42333CB00026B/3231